The Heart Attack Recovery Plan

The Heart Attack Recovery Plan

David Symes

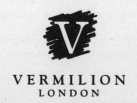

VERMILION
LONDON

Dedication

This book is dedicated to Michael Weeden, who died
on a sunny summer's day in 1995.

First published 1996

1 3 5 7 9 10 8 6 4 2

First published in the United Kingdom in 1996 by Vermilion
an imprint of Ebury Press
Random House UK Ltd
Random House, 20 Vauxhall Bridge Road, London SW1V 2SA

Random House Australia (Pty) Limited
20 Alfred Street, Milsons Point, Sydney, New South Wales 2061, Australia

Random House New Zealand Limited
18 Poland Road, Glenfield, Auckland 10, New Zealand

Random House South Africa (Pty) Limited
PO BOX 337, Bergvlei, South Africa

Random House UK Limited Reg. No. 954009

A CIP catalogue record for this book is available from the British Library

ISBN 0 09 181289 5

Typeset by Clive Dorman & Co.
Printed and bound in Great Britain by Mackays of Chatham plc

Papers used by Vermilion are natural, recyclable products made from wood
grown in sustainable forests.

Contents

Acknowledgements

During writing this book, help and advice have been received from many sources, the most important of which have been: Dr Tim Dudgeon, GP; Suzy Hopking, cardiac rehabilitation nurse; Kevin Power; Alan Stone; Sujata Bristow, medical herbalist; Dr Peter Travis; Rachel Hosken, cardiac rehabilitation nurse; Rod Lamb, fitness consultant; Andy Westwood, leisure centre manager; Barbara Fison, cardiac rehabilitation nurse; Dr David Hanratty, GP; Dr Hugh Carling, retired GP; Dr John Dean, cardiologist; Dr Brian Steggles, GP; Catherine Peel of the cardiac rehabilitation department at the British Heart Foundation; Dr Hugh Bethell of the British Association for Cardiac Rehabilitation; Helen Stokes of the British Association for Cardiac Rehabilitation; Cindy Cull, aerobics teacher; Jenny Bell, exercise physiologist; Di Allaker, of the Physical Activity Programme of Southern Buckinghamshire Health Promotion Department; Dr Bob Lewin, *Heart Manual* coordinator; Linley Dodd, nutritionist; Eric Hodges. My thanks go to all these individuals. The section in Chapter 10 on eating out is based on valuable material supplied by the Family Heart Association.

Dr Richard Wray, consultant cardiologist at the Conquest Hospital, St Leonards on Sea, and Dr John Dean, consultant cardiologist at the Royal Devon and Exeter Hospital, Exeter, have both been through the manuscript and advised influentially on a number of changes and amendments.

I must also thank Sarah Sutton, editor and publisher at Vermilion, whose idea this first was and who has encouraged and supported me during the research and writing that has occurred over the last few months.

David Symes
October 1995

1 Introduction

If you stopped a random assortment of people in the street and asked them what was the number one killer disease in this country, the majority of people would probably tell you that it is cancer. For various reasons, cancer has taken hold of the public's imagination; it has become a latter day bogeyman, lurking around the corner, waiting to pounce on you. To be sure, cancer does get a lot of media attention, as campaigns are launched to raise awareness of one sort of cancer or a new treatment is announced as having some effectiveness against another cancer.

But cancer isn't the major killer in the UK, even if you add together all the deaths from all the different sorts of cancer. AIDS isn't the major killer, despite its notoriety. Nor is it car accidents.

Heart disease – the epidemic

The disease that kills the most people in the UK each year is the furring up and blockage of the arteries that supply blood to the heart itself. In medical terms this translates as coronary heart disease or coronary artery disease, but whatever you call it the result is the same – angina if you're lucky, a mild heart attack if you're not so lucky and a massive fatal heart attack if you're unlucky.

The statistics are overwhelming. In 1991, coronary heart disease caused more than a quarter of all deaths in the UK. In the early 1990s about 170,000 people a year died of heart attacks; that's nearly 500 a day, or one every two to three minutes. And it's not a disease confined merely to men: women are almost as likely to die from it. Within the UK population, one in three men and one in four women will die of coronary heart disease. The disease mops up 2.5 per cent of the total National Health Service expenditure and is responsible for 35 million lost working days each year. It can be likened to a veritable epidemic.

A lot of publicity is nowadays given to the various changes you can make to your life that will help stave off the onset of heart disease. Perhaps the most publicity is given to diet. The food industry is making a fortune out of low-fat or no-fat alternatives to high-fat foods; people are encouraged to eat fruit and vegetables, to eat more white meat and fish and less red meat and processed meats; bookshop shelves are groaning under the weight of low-fat diet books, high-fibre diet books, raw-food diet books. And if you want to lose weight, you could buy a book a week and only scratch the surface of the advice that is available.

Similarly, although to a lesser extent, the benefits of exercise in preventing the onset of heart disease are publicised. First it was jogging, then distance running, then aerobics, then high-impact and low-impact aerobics, then step aerobics, then aerobic trampolining. Now there's boxercise, skipping, aqua-aerobics, powerwalking – the list grows ever larger. If you go into any leisure centre, you'll find that the range of classes and activities available is enormous, while in the bookshops yet more shelves are groaning under the weight of 'How to do it' exercise books by trim, slim (and fabulously rich) celebrities.

Ironically, the greatest impact on the onset of of heart disease can be made by giving up smoking, yet you'll find very few books, and even fewer courses, on how to give up smoking. What little publicity that is given to this course of action seems to have reached a plateau in its effectiveness and among young people smoking is now on the increase, which has serious implications for the future.

But what impact have these diets and fitness routines, the cholesterol awareness and emphasis on aerobic exercise, had on the health of the nation? Well, to be honest, not a lot. Since the Second World War Great Britain has been close to the top of the league table in the incidence of deaths from coronary heart disease and the situation has hardly changed over recent years. That the situation *can* be changed has been shown by the positions of other countries in the league table. Other Western industrialised countries, such as the US, Australia and New Zealand, have managed to reduce their incidence of deaths from coronary heart disease and have moved down the table, while countries in the former Eastern Bloc that are now beginning to share in the affluence of the West are shooting up the table. Perhaps the most significant change can be seen in countries like Japan. Time was when the Japanese ate a diet rich in fish and vegetables and low in fat, and lived a traditional agricultural life; then, heart disease was hardly known in their country. Gradually Western ways began to permeate their culture – Western food, Western cigarettes, a Western lifestyle – and, concomitantly, heart disease has become more and more of a problem.

• • •

What if you have heart disease?

But what we have looked at so far is what we can do to limit the onset of coronary heart disease. What happens if you have already had a heart attack or suffer from heart disease or angina? Are you going to have to 'take it easy' for the rest of your life, 'not overdo it'? Are you always going to be viewed as someone who is somehow not well?

Well, the simple answer is that there is a lot that you and your family can do to help you to recover successfully. There is nothing to stop someone who has had a heart attack or who suffers from angina from making a complete recovery, and perhaps gaining a far greater level of health and fitness than they had before the incident of heart disease.

This book aims to give sensible and practical advice on what you and your family can do to achieve these goals:

- It explains what the heart is and what it does.
- It explains what heart disease is, what the risk factors are and what you can do to reduce these risks.
- It explains exactly what a heart attack is – what happens and what it feels like.
- It explains what happens to you when you go into hospital after a heart attack, and what medical and surgical treatment you might receive.
- It explains what is involved in the recovery process, in hospital, once you get home and over the longer term.
- It explains what you and your family can do to ensure that you make the best possible recovery.
- It details what rehabilitation programmes may be available to you and what you can do if there are none in your area.
- It gives an insight into the psychological processes that might come into play during your recovery period and how you might deal with them.

If you have had a heart attack or suffer from angina, it is not the end of the world. Look upon it as a warning – if you continue living life as you have been, you leave yourself liable to further damage from coronary heart disease. But if you heed the warning and take it upon yourself to address the underlying causes of the heart disease, you can minimise your risk and at the same time probably lead a much happier and healthier life than you had before the heart attack.

The decision is yours, but there is a lot of help available. This book will add considerably to your ability to help yourself and will ensure that you know how best to use the help that others can provide.

2 Understanding heart disease

The heart

- 'My heart aches with love for you.'
- 'I love you with all my heart.'
- 'You are my heart's desire.'
- 'I'm broken-hearted.'
- 'My heart was in my mouth.'
- 'I learned it by heart.'
- 'His heart wasn't in it.'
- 'You must take this lesson to heart.'
- 'She cried her heart out.'
- 'We must have a heart to heart talk.'
- 'Take heart, it's not that bad.'
- 'He put his heart and soul into his work.'
- 'My heart sank when I saw what had happened.'
- 'He wore his heart on his sleeve.'

We could go on, ad infinitum, adding to this list of common phrases that involve reference to the heart. However, even with this brief list, it should be easy to see that the heart is something that we perceive as being at the very centre of our being, something vital, something essential, an organ of strength and sensitivity. Yet what exactly is the heart, this organ on which we depend so much? What does it do?

To begin with, we must go back to basics. Nearly all the organs and tissues of the body – the muscles and brain cells, liver and kidneys, eyes and ears, for example – need oxygen to function, just as a car engine needs oxygen for the petrol to work. Air containing oxygen is taken into the lungs, from where it passes into the bloodstream and is then transported around the body to where it is needed. All these organs and tissues also need food – nutrients or fuel – in order to work, and these are also transported in the bloodstream. Waste products have to be removed from cells, tissues and organs – another task for the bloodstream. And many functions of the immune system are carried

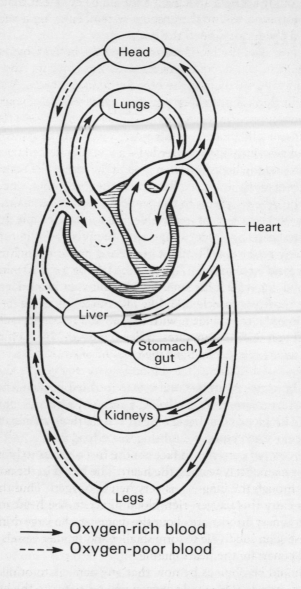

Fig. 1 *The blood circulation system.*

out by constituents of the bloodstream as they circulate around the body. From this brief catalogue, it should be apparent that the bloodstream forms an essential transport system, carrying a wide range of cells and chemicals around the body.

But how does the blood move around the body? Obviously it can't just dribble its way around. It needs some sort of pump. And that's what the heart does – it pumps the blood around the body. A simple task, you might think. But to keep pumping every second of your life, lifting the equivalent of 10 tons (10 tonnes) of blood 100 miles (160 km) over the course of a lifetime? It's a tall order. If you were to approach an engineer and describe what was needed – a four-chambered pump to pump blood around the lungs and then around the rest of the body – he could probably draw up a design. But if you then said that, once installed, there would be no access to the pump for repair and maintenance, he would write the job off as impossible. But for most people that's exactly what the heart does – it pumps away happily for a lifetime without giving any problems. Think of clenching and unclenching your fist every second for a minute. Then think of doing for it 10 minutes. Then think of doing it for a lifetime. That's what your heart does.

The heart is a muscle and, like all muscles, it needs its own blood supply in order to provide it with oxygen and nutrients and to remove the waste products it generates. Indeed, it needs a very efficient blood supply, when you think about the amount of work it has to do during the course of a lifetime. The blood vessels that supply the heart are called the *coronary arteries and veins*, so called because they encircle the heart like a corona or crown. The coronary arteries supply the heart muscle with blood containing oxygen and nutrients, while the coronary veins remove the blood containing waste products.

The coronary arteries in fact are the first arteries to branch off the aorta, or main artery leaving the heart. The blood in the aorta has just passed through the lungs, so is very rich in oxygen. Thus the coronary arteries carry this oxygen-rich blood direct to the heart muscle. The larger coronary arteries are about the diameter of a large drinking straw, but these soon subdivide to form smaller and smaller vessels that encircle and penetrate the heart muscle.

It should be obvious by now that any damage to or disease of the coronary arteries that supply oxygen and nutrients to the heart muscle is going to have potentially disastrous results. If the heart is not supplied effectively with oxygen and nutrients it is going to function less and less efficiently, blood will be pumped to the rest of the body less effectively, the heart will start to complain when it is overloaded and it will become overloaded increasingly frequently. In short, we have coronary heart disease – disease caused by the less efficient functioning of the coronary arteries of the heart.

Problems with the heart

There are many problems that can assail the heart. The heart has to be electrically stimulated by the nervous system in order to beat regularly and difficulties can arise in the regularity or transmission of these signals. The heart can become infected by germs – bacteria or viruses.

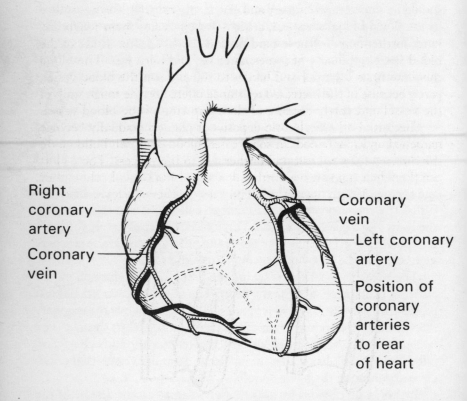

Right coronary artery

Coronary vein

Coronary vein

Left coronary artery

Position of coronary arteries to rear of heart

Fig. 2 *The blood vessels serving the heart.*

The valves in the heart can start to misfunction, either due to infection or degeneration. However, in this book we are concerned with one underlying problem, and that is *atherosclerosis*, or a furring up of the arteries, and in particular a furring up of the arteries that supply the heart with oxygen and nutrients – the coronary arteries.

Atherosclerosis

The word 'atherosclerosis' is quite a mouthful, but is very easy to understand as long as you remember that it is made up of two Greek words: *athere*, meaning 'porridge' or 'gruel', and *scleros*, meaning hard. Atherosclerosis, then, is a hard porridgey-looking deposit that is found embedded on the walls of the arteries. The walls of the blood vessels should be smooth and slippery and elastic, offering the least resistance to the flow of blood. Instead, atherosclerosis makes them rough and hard; furthermore, as these hard deposits build up, the inside of the blood vessel gradually becomes narrower and narrower. The blood therefore finds it harder and harder to travel down the blood vessel, partly because of the increased resistance offered by the rough walls of the vessel and partly because of the narrowing of the blood vessel.

The initial atherosclerotic deposits or plaques gradually become hardened and toughened. In some cases, blood clots can build up on the surface of the deposit and further add to the process. These clots can then detach and travel further down the blood vessel, where they may become lodged against other plaques of atherosclerosis, with the

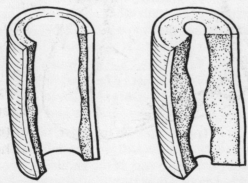

Fatty deposit
begins to build up

Several years later the
blood flow is nearly blocked

Fig. 3 *Build up of atherosclerotic deposits in the arteries gradually blocks the blood flow.*

risk that they will block the blood vessel. In general, though, the usual cause of a heart attack with heart muscle damage is where deposits or plaques rupture and scabs then form on the surface and builds up, blocking off the blood vessel completely.

The overall result is that a small cholesterol-rich scabby fibrous bulge appears in the artery wall, partially blocking off the artery and causing turbulence where there should be smooth efficient blood flow. The atherosclerosis can cause a weakness in the artery that may eventually rupture within the artery. As we have seen, it may produce a complete blockage of the blood vessel, either directly or because a piece of the deposit breaks free and lodges somewhere else.

Atherosclerosis can occur anywhere in the arteries in any part of the body, the resulting disease depending on the site of the problem:

- In the brain it can cause a stroke.
- It can cause poor vision.
- It can cause kidney failure.
- If the legs are affected it can cause pain, lameness and even gangrene.

But it is the effect that atherosclerosis has on the coronary arteries, the arteries that supply the heart, that is most critical. The furring up process takes place slowly and insidiously, and the coronary arteries are able to compensate up to a point by linking up and developing parallel branches of the vessels. It also appears that the heart can cope with some diminution in its supply of oxygen and nutrients. However, these compensatory mechanisms can only work up to a point; beyond that point you will start to notice the symptoms of coronary heart disease:

- Angina.
- Heart attack, that may or may not be fatal.

Angina
Angina is a warning, a cry for help from the heart, telling the sufferer that all is not well. It can manifest itself in a number of forms of discomfort, depending on the severity of the problem:
- A tightness or band around the chest.
- A gripping pain in the chest.
- A feeling of oppression in the chest – 'It settled like a moth on my heart, and closed around it'.
- A feeling of uselessness in the arms.

- Pain in the arms, especially the left arm, that may run down to the wrist and hand.
- Pain in the neck and chin.
- Breathlessness.

When describing it, the sufferer often places a hand or clenched fist on the middle of the chest, or both hands are placed on the lower chest.

Angina is usually brought on by exertion – when the heart has extra demands made of it, usually during bouts of exercise or hard work – and is likely to be worse after a meal, when walking up hill, walking against a wind and on cold days.

- 'Going up even a mild slope brought on the pain.'
- 'I couldn't even walk up four steps without becoming painfully breathless and my chest tightening.'

If you continue with the exercise or work, the pain, discomfort and distress usually get worse, although some people can 'work it off'. Usually the pain and discomfort are so bad that the thought of doing anything other than keeping still is out of the question. After a few minutes, maybe 10 minutes, of rest, the pain and distress wear off.

What happens is that the coronary arteries that are partially blocked by atherosclerosis cannot get enough oxygen and nutrients to the heart muscle to cope with the extra demands that are being placed on the heart. The body responds by producing the symptoms of angina, effectively stopping you from asking the heart to do something that it is no longer capable of. You stop exerting yourself, the heart's need for extra oxygen is gradually reduced, and the pain and discomfort go away.

The early symptoms of angina may be comparatively mild and initially the individual may do nothing about them. As they get worse, though, sooner or later there will be a tendency to go to see their GP, who may in turn refer them on to the cardiology department at the local general hospital (although it has to be added that many people who suffer from angina do not go and see any doctor). Tests will be undertaken to determine the severity of the problem, drugs may be prescribed, and advice will be given on giving up smoking if necessary, taking more exercise, changing the diet and weight loss if necessary. Providing the advice is heeded, it may be that nothing more needs to be done and the problem recedes. The lifestyle changes need to be long-term and permanent, though, if the problem is not to recur – and this is a message that will be repeated throughout this book.

In some cases it may be necessary to deal with the furred-up coronary arteries in a more drastic manner, either by angioplasty or coronary artery bypass surgery (both detailed later in the book, see pp56, 82). These interventions will certainly relieve the symptoms of angina, but if the more fundamental problems – smoking, lack of exercise, poor diet, obesity – are not addressed, the symptoms are likely to recur sooner or later.

Some people suffer from what is known as *unstable angina*, whereby the symptoms of angina come on at any time of the day or night and are not related to exertion or stress. This is a far more serious problem, suggesting that the coronary arteries are very seriously diseased, and will raise the probability of angioplasty or surgery.

Heart attack

Heart attack is the layman's term for what the medical world describes as a *myocardial infarction* (abbreviated to MI) or an *acute myocardial infarction* (or a *cardiac event*), and this medical term is an extremely clear description of what happens. *Infarction* means the death of an area of tissue caused by the blocking of the blood circulation and the *myocardium* is the heart muscle; an MI is therefore the death of an area of the heart muscle due to the blockage of its blood supply.

A heart attack is usually brought on when a coronary artery with atherosclerosis suffers from a rupture to a plaque; a clot forms where the rupture has occurred and this causes a blockage to the blood vessel. The blockage may only be temporary, and the heart attack be so mild as to go unnoticed, although it will almost invariably show up in subsequent tests. More serious blockages will produce the classic symptoms of a heart attack:

- The same sort of pain as is experienced with angina – a tightness or band around the chest; a gripping pain in the chest; a feeling of oppression in the chest; pain in the arms, especially the left arm, that may run down to the wrist and hand; pain in the neck and chin. At its worst this pain can be the most severe ever experienced.
- A feeling of indigestion, often not associated with eating anything out of the ordinary like a large meal; the great majority of patients describe and truly believe they have indigestion.
- A feeling of uselessness in one or both arms.
- Tingling in the fingers, especially the ring and little fingers.
- Nausea and vomiting.
- Breathlessness.

- Exhaustion.
- Feeling clammy and sweaty.
- Looking pale, grey or even slightly bluish around the face.
- Feeling 'odd', 'peculiar', 'strange', 'dizzy'.

The speed with which these symptoms develop will vary, depending on how much of the heart muscle is affected by the blockage to its blood supply. At its worst, the heart attack results in sudden death – in one in five people this shows up as the first, and final, presentation of coronary heart disease. Usually, though, the symptoms develop gradually and to begin with the sufferer may attempt to continue with what they are doing, occasionally for a period of hours or longer. The most common heart attack, though, is serious enough for the health service to be called within minutes and, as we shall see later, the speed with which the services can be mobilised is critical.

A heart attack invariably leads to a period in hospital, during which the risk of a subsequent heart attack or associated heart failure from other causes are as far as possible dealt with and removed. There is then a recovery period in hospital, a recovery period at home and, ideally, a subsequent rehabilitation programme that slowly but surely increases the stamina of the heart muscle. It is this period of recovery and rehabilitation that we then will be concentrating on in this book,

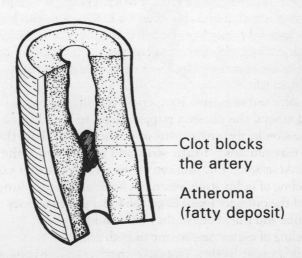

Clot blocks the artery

Atheroma (fatty deposit)

Fig. 4 *A heart attack is caused when a blood clot blocks a furred-up coronary artery.*

helping you to make the most of it and, if necessary, to devise your own rehabilitation programme.

The severity of a heart attack will very much depend on the amount of heart muscle involved. If a large area has been damaged by the heart attack, then the individual has to understand that their heart will not be able to work as efficiently as it once did, and that they are going to have to accept limits to the amount of activity that they can manage. However, for most people who have a heart attack the damaged area is small, and there is no reason why they cannot return to a level of health, activity and fitness that they had before their heart attack.

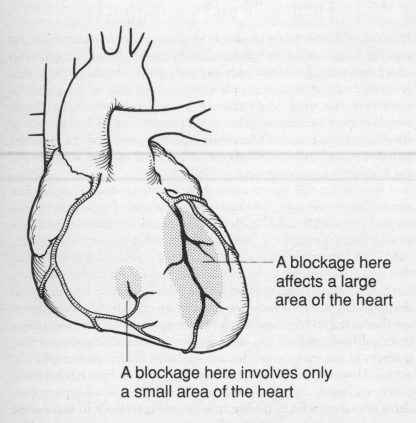

A blockage here affects a large area of the heart

A blockage here involves only a small area of the heart

Fig. 5 A blockage at the end of a coronary artery will not cause much damage to the heart muscle. A blockage near the beginning of a coronary artery will shut off the blood supply to a much larger area of the heart muscle.

Even those who have suffered the most severe heart attacks can ensure that they make the most of the situation they find themselves in. But for everyone who has suffered from heart disease – and this applies as much to people with angina as it does to those who have experienced heart attacks – the recovery and rehabilitation have to involve fundamental changes in their lives that address the risk of further incidents of heart disease, and that increase their fitness and stamina levels. These changes are easily achievable, but they are fundamental, and they have to be permanent, and that is perhaps the most important message of this book.

Heartache and heart attacks

Much is spoken and written about the connections between the mind and the body – how one's behaviour, personality and thoughts can affect the workings of one's body and one's state of health. I think that it is fair to say that most people would accept that in some way, in some part, the mind does influence the body and vice versa. Some people dispute this, arguing that it is an impossible link to prove and therefore doesn't exist. Others state that the mind and the body are indivisible, and that the well-being of the mind and the well-being of the body are one and the same.

I raise this point here because there are those who maintain that symptoms, incidents of ill-health, reflect features of the psychology of the individual – for example, that a heart attack is related in some way to some event or aspect of life that strikes 'at the heart' of that individual. Perhaps it is something that is obvious, perhaps it is something that occurred long ago and has been internalised for many years. I am not prepared to pass an opinion on these ideas; anyone who gives any deep thought to a serious disease that has affected them is sometime or another going to have to consider these matters. This is ostensibly a practical book on how you can best recover from the serious consequences of coronary heart disease – a heart attack and, implicitly, angina. However, as I have already stated, to recover from heart disease, to recover health and energy, and to reduce the risk of subsequent incidents of coronary heart disease, you are going to have to make some permanent changes to your life. These changes are not necessarily difficult, but some of them are fundamental and they must be permanent. Such changes are bound to have an effect on your mood and personality. For example, at the simplest level, it is harder to feel miserable when you are fit and healthy and taking exercise than when you are unfit, unhealthy and take no exercise.

If you want to investigate or address the links between the psychology of the individual and the onset of a heart attack, there are many paths you can follow. All that is offered in this book is practical advice and guidance on how best to recover from a heart attack. However, it may be that if you choose to make the most of rehabilitation and recovery, and gain a level of health and fitness that perhaps you have not known for some time, some deeper problems might also be addressed along the way.

Finally

There are some essential facts that you must recognise, that you must remember as you work your way through this book and that you must keep in mind as you recover from your heart attack. Learn these facts; make certain your family and friends learn them. They are the bedrock of an optimism that you need in order to maximise your recovery.

- The first day or two after a heart attack is when you are most at risk of another heart attack or, more likely, when the electrics to the heart go haywire and stops beating properly. Both can be dealt with in the cardiac/coronary care unit. After two days these risks diminish rapidly.
- The heart has a tremendous ability to recover from a heart attack. After a week it is usually working just as well as it used to.
- During a heart attack an area of the heart muscle is damaged. In a couple of weeks this damaged area scars over. Scar tissue is tough – stronger than ordinary tissue.
- The heart adjusts to having a bit of scar tissue in it – the remaining muscle takes up the extra work, usually without any problems.
- You will feel weak and tired after a heart attack. Partly it's the shock, partly it's lying in bed doing nothing – your body goes out of condition very quickly. If you make the effort to get going again, and follow the suggestions for exercise and activity, you will quickly lose the feeling of tiredness and feebleness.
- If you sit around doing very little after a heart attack, whether it's in hospital or when you get home, you increase your risk of another heart attack. You should be doing a bit more each day, gradually building up your exercise and activity levels.

3 Are you at risk?

What does being at risk mean?

Heart attacks and angina are caused by coronary heart disease, and coronary heart disease is in turn caused by atherosclerosis – the furring up of the arteries supplying the heart muscle – compounded by thrombosis or blood clots. This is a simple statement, but it begs a number of questions that are not at all easy to answer and that have led to a number of differences of opinion within the medical world.

For example, what causes this furring up of the coronary arteries? This is a simple question, but there is no simple answer to it. Even to state that there is a number of interrelated causes of atherosclerosis is a gross simplification. At the end of the day, no one can tell you that if you do this or don't do that you will definitely develop coronary heart disease and have a heart attack. Certainly our knowledge and understanding of cause and effect in the development of atherosclerosis and coronary heart disease are improving, but there are still large areas of uncertainty where statements and advice have to be hedged around with ifs and buts.

What we do have, though, is the concept of a risk factor. This is a statistical concept that predicts the chance of something happening or not happening. For example, if you smoke you have a higher risk of suffering from coronary heart disease (and many other diseases for that matter) than someone who does not smoke, and that increased risk can be quantified depending on how long you have smoked and how many you smoke per day. But be careful to note that this is not the same as saying that smoking causes heart disease. Doubtless we all know of someone who smoked 40 a day all their lives and lived to the age of 91 before being run over by a bus. That they didn't die of heart disease, or any other smoking-related problems, at a much younger age is because they were in the small section of the smoking population who are predicted not to die of a smoking-related illness.

So how is a risk factor assessed? First of all, you obviously need a

23

hypothesis, an idea, to test. For example, it is observed that choles-terol is a major constituent of the atherosclerotic plaque that furs up the arteries in coronary heart disease. Your conclusion might therefore be that high cholesterol levels in the blood can increase the chance of coronary heart disease, because the cholesterol is likely to become incorporated in the atherosclerotic matter furring up the arteries. To test this hypothesis you take two similar groups of people, one with high blood cholesterol levels and the other with low blood cholesterol levels, and you follow them over a period of years and count the number in each group who die of coronary heart disease. You might therefore be satisfied when you find that over 10 years, say, more people from the group with high blood cholesterol levels died of coronary heart disease than from the group with low blood cholesterol levels. Wonderful, you might think; this goes to prove conclusively that people with high blood cholesterol levels have a higher chance of dying from coronary heart disease than people with low blood cholesterol, and therefore a raised blood cholesterol level is a risk factor.

But is it? Perhaps the group with high cholesterol levels included a disproportionate number of smokers. Did you take account of this fact? Can you tell that it wasn't the smoking that caused the disease? Maybe the smoking caused the high cholesterol levels. Or maybe the group with low cholesterol levels included a disproportionate number of women. Do women have a low risk of coronary heart disease because they are women or do they have a naturally low cholesterol level? How much exercise did the members of the two groups take? Were any of them left-handed?

In fact it has been shown by various studies that a high blood cholesterol level does lead to a high risk of coronary heart disease, but you should begin to understand that it far from simple establishing what the risk factors are for coronary heart disease. And working out how serious is the risk attached to each factor is even more of a mine-field. As already stated, although certain truths have become apparent in recent years, this is still an area of some debate and controversy within the medical establishment.

What are the risk factors?

In this section we will look at the principal factors that put you at increased risk of suffering from coronary heart disease and therefore of having a heart attack or angina.

Family

If you are having a medical examination to assess your risk of coronary heart disease, one of the first questions you will be asked will be about your family members, your parents and grandparents. Did any of your parents or grandparents have heart attacks or other symptoms of coronary heart disease? Did any of them die of a heart attack? Any of your uncles or aunts? Any brothers or sisters? At what age?

The answers to these questions will help to establish whether or not you come from a family that is prone to coronary heart disease. If you do, then risks from other factors need to be taken more seriously and addressed more strongly.

Why some families are more at risk of coronary heart disease is still poorly understood. There are some families where there is a congenital problem (a problem they are born with and inherit) with their fat metabolism and they have very high levels of cholesterol in their blood; as a high blood cholesterol level is a risk in itself, this means that the members of the family are at high risk of coronary heart disease from a very early age, often suffering heart attacks as young as their 20s or 30s. In other families, though, the reasons for the high incidence of deaths from heart attack are far from clear. Anyone from such a family has to accept that increased risk, without there being a clear explanation available at the moment. What they can do is address the other risk factors over which they do have some control.

Age

Age is another risk factor over which you have no control. As you get older, from adolescence onwards, your risk of suffering from coronary heart disease increases. The most rapid increase in risk is for men during the period from 40 to 60 years of age and for women from 50 to 60 years (see page 26 for an explanation of the discrepancy between men and women). This is not to say that men between 40 and 60 are most at risk of a heart attack. What it means is that the greatest increase in risk for a man occurs between 40 and 60; before 40 and after 60 the risk is still increasing with age, but not nearly so fast.

Heart disease

It may seem like stating the obvious, but if you have already had problems with coronary heart disease – angina or perhaps a heart attack – you are at increased risk of suffering from coronary heart disease. Put simply, if you already have coronary heart disease you are likely to continue to suffer from it.

The major point of this book is to provide assistance and back-up in order to help you return to full health and activity after a heart attack. However, a parallel aim is to help you reduce your risks of suffering from further heart attacks or angina. If you have already suffered a heart attack or angina you should see it as essential to your future health and well-being that you reduce any subsequent risk of the same thing recurring, and in part this is what this book aims to do.

Sex

Many people are under the impression that women very rarely suffer from angina and heart attacks. Nothing could be further from the truth. In the UK one in three men die from coronary heart disease; for women the incidence is one in four. This book is not just for men: it is for men *and* women.

Somehow the female sex hormones that circulate in a woman's bloodstream between puberty and the menopause provide protection against coronary heart disease. However, once a woman has passed her menopause and the production of these hormones is reduced, this protection is removed and her risk of suffering from angina or a heart attack starts to catch up with that of men, although at no time does it overtake it.

Smoking

If a company were to try and launch a new product made from the the leaves of a plant that were dried, shredded, treated with chemicals and then packed into thin paper tubes so that it could be smoked, a myriad of questions would be raised.

'Why would anyone want to inhale smoke? Normally people avoid smoke.'

'Ah, but they'll enjoy it because the leaves contain a stimulant.'

'But won't they get bored with it after a time?'

'Maybe, but the stimulant is very addictive and once they start they won't be able to stop. We'll have a captive market.'

'Well... er, OK. But apart from the addiction, are there any other problems?'

'Well, yes, there are some small health problems – cancer, breathing difficulties, heart disease, and a few others – but nothing the public won't be able to cope with.'

What chance would there be of any such product being allowed anywhere near the public?

Unfortunately, cigarettes are a fact of life. That smoking poses a risk to health is generally accepted, although most people would be surprised at the range of illnesses it can give rise to and the overall scale of the problem. For example, did you know that smoking is the most important cause of avoidable death – about 110,000 deaths a year – in Great Britain? This is about six times as many as caused by accidents, murder, suicide and AIDS *put together*.

Smoking is a very serious risk factor for coronary heart disease. People who smoke more than 20 cigarettes a day have over double the risk of coronary heart disease of non-smokers and it takes up to 10 years of non-smoking for a reformed smoker's risk to drop to that of a permanent non-smoker of similar age, although the reduction in risk becomes apparent from very early after the smoker quits.

Smoking is much more of a risk factor for coronary heart disease than being overweight, so if someone tells you that they don't want to stop smoking because they'll put on weight, you can point this out as the nonsense it is.

Women who smoke are creating even greater problems for themselves than they might at first realise. As we have seen, before the menopause women are protected against the risks of coronary heart disease by the female sex hormones that circulate in their bloodstream; after the menopause the levels of these hormones diminish, as does the protection against heart disease conferred by them. Smoking somehow seems to bring on the age of menopause earlier, so not only does smoking add its own risks as regards coronary heart disease, but for women it also appears to remove their natural protection against risk at an earlier age.

Exercise

Despite the fact that the interest in exercise and personal fitness have spawned major industries, as a nation we take far too little exercise. Indeed, it would be true to say that the sedentary western way of life is to blame for many of the ills that we are now prone to. It is only within the last couple of generations that this inactivity has become a way of life. Before then there was far more manual work, much less private transport, and people expected to have to take a lot of exercise as part of their daily routine. This is one reason why rates of heart disease were much lower earlier in the century. Even as recently as a generation ago, most schoolchildren would be expected to take reasonable and obvious periods of exercise, whether as part of their everyday active lives or as part of their school day. A recent study, however, that measured young teenagers' heart rates over a week was unable, in many cases, to detect any incidents of raised heart rate, even during school periods of sport or PE. Inactive children will in most cases grow up to be inactive adults, so it appears that the seeds of many health problems are already with us by the time people reach early adulthood.

Strictly speaking, lack of exercise is not a risk factor: rather, it is the taking of exercise that is a protective factor against coronary heart disease, roughly equivalent to not smoking or not having high blood pressure or high blood cholesterol levels. It is a complex picture, though, because taking exercise also modifies other risk factors: it can lower blood pressure, it can favourably modify blood cholesterol levels and can help in reducing obesity.

Cholesterol level

There has been much controversy over the links between blood cholesterol levels and risk of coronary heart disease. This has given rise to some major investigations into these links and the picture is somewhat clearer now, although it is still true to say that the medical world places varying degrees of emphasis on the results of these investigations.

As an overall conclusion one can say simply that for every 1 per cent that the blood cholesterol level is raised, there is a 2 per cent increase in the risk of coronary heart disease, although in fact a high cholesterol level tends to cause an even higher risk of coronary heart disease. Cholesterol is transported in the bloodstream in a number of carriers known as *lipoproteins*. From the point of view of risk of coronary heart disease, the two most significant lipoproteins are low-density lipoprotein and high-density lipoprotein, mercifully abbreviated to LDL and HDL. LDL cholesterol appears to be involved in incorporating cholesterol into the deposits in the arteries that cause the furring-up process in coronary heart disease. In contrast, HDL appears to be involved in the reverse process. In simple terms, therefore, HDL can be seen as Good Thing, or protective against coronary heart disease, while LDL can be seen as a Bad Thing, or a risk factor for coronary heart disease.

Many people assume that their blood cholesterol level is directly associated with the amount of cholesterol they take in in their diet and ruthlessly examine every item of food they buy for the quantities of cholesterol that they might contain. In fact the blood cholesterol level is directly linked with the amount of *fat* we consume, particularly with the amount of saturated fat. As a gross generalisation, we all eat too much fat, we all eat too much saturated fat, and as a result, as a population, we all have high blood cholesterol levels – about two-thirds of the UK population has a blood cholesterol level above what is generally recommended by the medical world.

But what is this generally recommended level? Blood cholesterol levels are measured in units called millimoles per litre, abbreviated to mmol/l. What exactly these units are is not important here. What are important are the figures themselves. In general:

- Below 5.2 mmol/l is the ideal. If you have other risk factors such as smoking, obesity or high bood pressure, you should be advised by your GP to do something about them, but in general if you have a cholesterol level below 5.2 you will be sent on your way with a smile.
- Between 5.2 and 6.4 mmol/l is seen as a mild problem. You should be advised on healthy eating and exercise, as well as on any other risk factors you may have. You should heed this advice.
- Between 6.5 and 7.8 mmol/l is seen as a more serious problem, and advice on diet, exercise and other risk factors for coronary heart disease should be more emphatic and detailed. Underlying causes of the problem should be sought by your doctor and addressed.
- Over 7.8 mmol/l is a severe problem and should be addressed with specialist advice, perhaps involving a dietitian and appointments at a lipid clinic.

If the cholesterol level is over 6.5 mmol/l you may be given what is known as a fasting cholesterol test, which will give the figures for HDL and LDL:

- The LDL level should be as low as possible, preferably under 5 mmol/l.
- The HDL level should be as high as possible, and preferably over 1 mmol/l.

Your blood cholesterol level is usually assessed by testing a small sample of blood that is withdrawn from a vein in your arm. This sample is then sent off to a laboratory, and the result comes back a day or so later. There are now also a range of machines available that can give you a reading of your total blood cholesterol level in a matter of minutes, using a pinprick blood sample, and you may come across such 'instant' cholesterol tests in situations where a doctor is not on hand to interpret the results or give follow-up advice; indeed, it is even possible to measure your own cholesterol level using a home testing kit. Such tests can be very useful in giving you an idea of what your level is, but it must be remembered that they are only as accurate as the person calibrating and operating the equipment, and should always be followed up with advice from a doctor and subsequent testing to confirm or add more detail to the initial result. If you have such a test, the advice is always to go and see your GP if you are in any way concerned or unsure about what it means.

Blood pressure

High blood pressure, known in the medical world as *hypertension*, appears to increase the formation of atherosclerotic deposits and is therefore a strong risk factor for coronary heart disease. Blood pressure is merely a measurement of the pressure exerted by the heart as it pumps blood around the body. It is usually measured by strapping a cuff round your upper arm and inflating this cuff until the blood supply is temporarily cut off; the pressure is then released, the blood supply gradually resumes, and the doctor or nurse uses a stethoscope to listen for certain sounds that indicate your blood pressure as measured on a tube of mercury or an electronic machine.

You will always see two blood pressure readings together, e.g. 120/70:

- The first is called the *systolic pressure*, and indicates the pressure exerted by the heart as it contracts and squeezes the blood out into the arteries. In the example above this is 120 mm Hg (short for milli-metres of mercury, although these units need not concern us here).
- The second number is called the *diastolic pressure*, and indicates the pressure in the blood system when the heart is relaxed and is filling with blood. In the example this is 70 mm Hg.

It is difficult to establish hard and fast rules for what is a desirable blood pressure. For a start, blood pressure tends to rise with age. However, the general rule is that the lower the blood pressure, the better (although if it is too low it can cause other problems, such as faintness on standing or getting out of bed). Systolic pressure – the first of the two readings – appears to be the better predictor of risk of coronary heart disease. A systolic pressure below 140 mm Hg is thought to be advisable, with a diastolic pressure below 90 mm Hg. If blood pressure is over 160/95, action certainly needs to be taken.

High blood pressure can also be a strong predictor of risk of strokes, kidney disease and eye problems. It has been estimated that a reduction in 6 to 8 mm Hg overall in the population, i.e. in the average blood pressure, could lead to a 25 per cent drop in the incidence of coronary heart disease in the population (and a 50 per cent reduction in the incidence of stroke).

Overweight

Many books on heart disease would probably head this section 'Obesity', which implies being seriously overweight. This is certainly not the same as being overweight; being overweight is merely being over a defined ideal weight for your height and sex. Various studies have demonstrated that there is a direct increase in one's risk of coronary heart disease with increase in weight above one's ideal weight. It is a far from simple story, though, as being overweight is often associated with high blood pressure and high blood cholesterol levels. (The latter should be self-evident; being overweight and a high blood cholesterol level both tend to be due to a high-fat diet.)

There are all sorts of tables and charts that can be used to determine whether or not you are overweight.

- The simplest merely correlate weight with height and state that if you are a man of such-and-such a height, then you ought to weigh so much.
- A more realistic assessment is to accept that there are bound to be variations in the population and to provide a chart that tells you for a given height what range of weight might indicate whether you are underweight, satisfactory, overweight or obese.
- Then there is a the body–mass index, or BMI (also known as the Quetelet index). This is recommended by many authorities as being the best indicator and for the mathematically minded is calculated by dividing one's weight (in kilograms) by one's height squared (as measured in metres). In practice, the BMI can most conveniently be measured from a chart and such a chart also usually indicates the relative risk of coronary heart disease associated with different levels of being overweight:
A BMI of 20 or less indicates being underweight.
A BMI of 20–5 indicates an acceptable level.

A BMI of 25–30 indicates being overweight, i.e. some health risk.
A BMI of 30–40 indicates obesity, i.e. moderate health risk.
A BMI of over 40 indicates severe obesity, i.e. high health risk.

- There is the waist circumference level. This has recently been established as action level 1 (37 inches [94 cm] in men and 31 inches [80 cm] in women) and action level 2 (40 inches [101 cm] for men and 34 inches [87 cm] for women). Below level 1 indicates a low risk of coronary heart disease while above level 2 indicates a high risk of coronary heart disease.

- Then there is the waist-to-hip ratio, i.e. the waist measurement divided by the hip measurement; if you have a waist of 38 inches (96 cm) and hips of 34 inches (86 cm) you have a ratio of 38/34, or just over 1. If you have a waist measurement of 30 inches and hips of 38 you have a ratio of 30/38, or considerably less than 1. A high waist:hip ratio is indicative of increased risk of coronary heart disease; for women 'high' is over 0.8, while for men it is over 1.

- A completely different assessment is to measure the thickness of a fold of skin. Above a certain thickness in a specific part of the body indicates that deposits of fat exist under the skin. As one loses weight, so this skin-fold will get thinner. (Although, if a person is also taking more exercise as well as losing weight, there may come a point where there is no more under-skin fat to be lost while the weight starts to increase slightly. This is because muscle is being added to the body and muscle is heavier than fat.)

Statistics show that about 45 per cent of the UK population is overweight and 14 per cent have a serious weight problem. Most people realise when they are overweight, although whether they admit this fact to other people, or even to themselves, is another matter.

If you are overweight you will undoubtedly already have received dietary advice from your GP, who should have impressed on you the risks attached to being overweight and made you aware of the limitations this extra weight is imposing on you. For example, if you are as much as 50 kg (8 stone) overweight you are having to carry around the equivalent of a sack of coal – up and down stairs, when you're doing the shopping, when you're at work. You can imagine the extra work that your body (including your heart) is having to do to cope with this burden.

Fortunately few of us are as much as overweight as this, but the sack of coal analogy can be quite a useful one to work with. Say you are

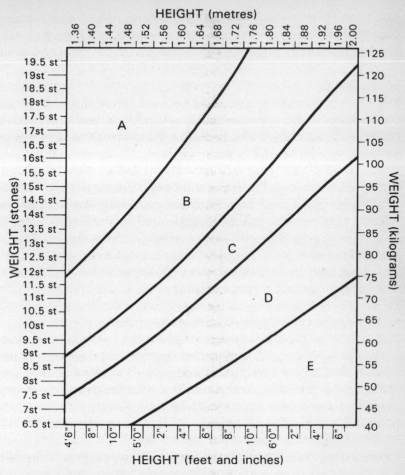

A Very obese - health is seriously at risk. Losing weight immediately is essential

B Obese - health is at risk. Losing weight now should be seriously considered

C Overweight - health could suffer. Some weight loss should now be considered

D Healthy - a desirable BMI figure indicating a healthy weight

E Underweight

Fig. 6 *Body–mass index chart.*

merely 10 kg (1½ stone) overweight; this is equivalent to carting around 10 bags of sugar. If you are 13 kg overweight (about 2 stone), this is as much as 13 bags of flour.

Ethnic groups

The UK population consists of various ethnic groups – Africans, Caribbeans, other Europeans, Asians. All these ethnic groups have various differences in health risks, but it has to be stated here that Asians have a higher risk of coronary heart disease than most other groups. Irrespective of their regional, cultural and religious differences, south Asians – Indians, Pakistanis and Bangladeshis – all have a significantly high risk of death from heart disease. At the moment this is a problem that is not satisfactorily addressed by the health service.

Personality types

Links have been drawn between personality types and the risk of coronary heart disease and subsequent heart attacks.

- Those with 'type A' personalities are competitive, always trying to do things better than anyone else, always trying to do as much as they possibly can. They almost choose to load themselves with stress, but are not very good at coping with it – they tend to lose their tempers easily, often have difficulty concentrating when they have a lot to do, are restless and fidgety.
- Type B personalities are far more relaxed, more easy going – they don't lose their tempers, don't make a drama out of a crisis. They may manage to get through just as much as a type A personality, but it never seems to be such an effort.

To many readers it may come as no surprise that type A personalities have been shown to be more at risk of coronary heart disease than type B personalities. However, it has to be said that the studies that show these links are not clearcut, and because of this many within the medical profession would pooh-pooh any links between personality and heart disease.

What is true is that if you react to stress by becoming anxious you produce a chemical called *adrenaline*. This is a very basic response and gives rise to what is know as the 'fight and flight' response. Back in prehistoric times any stress would probably have been life-threatening – for example, an attack – and this fight and flight response geared us up to do just that – stay and fight or run away as fast as possible. Today our stresses are more sophisticated and our responses have to be likewise; it is unacceptable to wallop the traffic warden who has just given you a parking ticket and running away would be considered most peculiar if you were asked an awkward question at a job interview.

The immediate response to this rush of adrenaline in the 'fight and flight' response is to increase the heart rate and to shut down many of the smaller arteries, which in turn raises the blood pressure, and to increase the levels of fat in the blood system. This is fine if we fight or run, actually making use of the resources that are mobilised, but if we don't we are left in a state of physical overexcitement, the heart placed under a burden, that may spill over into the next stressful challenge. Defusing this stress 'bomb' is therefore of importance.

It appears that those who can cope with the shocks and mental burden of late twentieth-century life without becoming stressed, anxious or tense are less at risk of coronary heart disease than are those who are tense, stressed out, constantly appearing to be hassled and under pressure. If possible, those type A personalities need to become more the relaxed type B personalities, although how easy this is is very hard to assess.

How to minimise your risk

This is not a detailed book on how to reduce your risks of coronary heart disease; it is a book on how best you can manage your recovery from a heart attack. Obviously, part of this recovery programme has to include the reduction of risk of another heart attack; to that end the chapters on food and exercise are perhaps the key chapters in this book.

This section merely takes a quick look at the general guidelines on how anyone can reduce their risk of coronary heart disease. It is a difficult area to deal with as the advice will vary from doctor to doctor, from book to book, from expert to expert. What is offered here is some commonsense advice that should be easy to understand and easy to act on. If you go and look at the more detailed advice, this section should allow you to understand what is being suggested.

Stop smoking
This is perhaps the most important single piece of advice you can have regarding any aspect of your health and well-being. Smoking is certainly the most important risk factor for coronary heart disease, but it is also

implicated in a host of other disease, including cancer (and here we are talking about a wide range of cancers – of the larynx, pharynx, mouth, gullet, pancreas, kidneys, bladder and stomach – not merely lung cancer) and respiratory diseases (diseases of the breathing system).

The advice is always, at all times:

- Not to start smoking.
- If you already smoke, give it up as soon as possible.

Now, this is very simple advice to give, but notoriously hard to act upon. If you do not smoke, there is a lot of pressure on you to start, particularly for young people – advertising, marketing images projected in all sorts of subtle and less-than-subtle ways, peer group pressure. Young people have never been better educated about the risks of smoking, yet smoking is on the increase amongst young people, particularly among girls, and as we have seen earlier in this chapter, women who smoke not only add to their risks of coronary heart disease but the smoking also brings on an earlier menopause, thus reducing the protection of the female sex hormones. This increase in young smokers says a lot about the power of advertising and marketing in shaping the way we behave.

Once you start smoking, you have to accept the fact that you become an addict, just like a heroin addict, and addictions are very difficult to give up. However, it can be done – millions have done it before and as our knowledge of addictive behaviour becomes more sophisticated, so more effective strategies for giving up smoking are developed. It is now accepted that it is not easy to give up smoking and that going back to smoking may be a stage in this process. It can be followed, however by another, bigger, effort to give up – this time perhaps for longer – perhaps to be followed by another relapse and another attempt. The relapses are not failures, merely stages along a road.

The most important thing is that you should want to give up smoking. It is not just a question of being told to give up smoking by your doctor, by your wife or husband, by your friends, by this book. You must understand the value in giving up smoking and really to want to give it up.

Strategies for giving up smoking are looked at in more depth later in the book. Many health areas can offer assistance if you want to give up – a specialised clinic or an adviser or self-help groups. Your GP or your health centre practice nurse can tell you if such assistance is available in your area.

Take more exercise

Again, a more detailed examination of the benefits of exercise and how exercise should play a key role in life of someone after a heart attack are looked at later in the book. Here is merely a look at how exercise can reduce everyone's risk of suffering from coronary heart disease in the first place.

We have already touched on the fact that we take less exercise than in the past. Most of us have cars, so there's no need to walk. Food is comparatively cheap, so there's no need to garden or grow your own fruit and veg. We all have TVs, so there's less inclination to go out and seek other forms of entertainment and activity. And we live in houses packed with labour-saving machines that remove much of the strenuous activity from everyday household life.

But what are the benefits of exercise? Why should it be so good at reducing your risk of coronary heart disease?

- It helps reduce some of the risk factors for coronary heart disease – cholesterol levels, body weight.
- It can certainly stop the furring-up process of the arteries to the heart and in some cases can reduce the existing furring-up.
- It can improve the blood supply to the heart muscle by encouraging cross-links between coronary arteries.
- The total volume of blood in the body is increased, as is its ability to transport oxygen to the muscles.
- The heart's stamina is improved, as is the body's. A greater physical workload can be tolerated by both.
- At a more subtle level, self-confidence is boosted and depression lifted.

That should be enough to be going on with, surely?

But what sort of exercise should you take? Well, the range is enormous, but we have to distinguish between those forms of exercise that are short-lived and sudden – that make you grunt! – and those that are longer-lasting and gradually make your heart beat faster and make you puff. The former include such activities as weight training and heavy digging; they are useful in strengthening specific groups of muscles, but do not help to improve stamina. The latter include such continuous forms of exercise as brisk walking, jogging, swimming and cycling, and the various forms of aerobics that are on offer in most adult education classes.

There are three important points to bear in mind if such exercise is to be of value in lowering your risk of coronary heart disease:

- There must be an increase in the beating of your heart and you must feel slightly out of breath – the two will tend to go together.
- Such exercise should take place at least three or four times a week.
- Such exercise should become a part of your life, for the rest of your life.

Walking is perhaps the most easily accessible form of exercise. You don't need special equipment or clothes and it can often be incorporated into the journey to work or to the shops. But bear in mind that although a stroll through the park with the dog is not to be decried, what we are talking about here is a brisk mile or two's walk with one stiffish hill along the way. At some point you should feel breathless. Chinese medicine has much advice to offer us in the West on how to stay healthy; one such piece of advice is that we should get breathless at least once every day.

As well as aiming to take up activities that involve exercise – swimming or cycling, for example – here are some simple ways you can introduce exercise into your day-to-day activities:

- You can walk to work, or to the train or to the shops or you can catch the bus a few stops further along the route.
- Walk the children to school – it will get them used to walking, as well as benefiting you.
- Use stairs instead of the lift or escalator.

Eat sensibly
Perhaps more has been written about and on the health benefits of different types of diet than on any other subject in popular medicine. Taken as a whole, the advice is often conflicting, sometimes misguided and occasionally dangerous. And always there is the emphasis on the word 'diet', the implication being that if you follow the advice you will be eating foods that others are not that you will be 'different' in some way or another.

The advice here is far from extreme. It is simple. It is simply to eat sensibly. As a nation we eat too much fat, we eat too little fruit and vegetables, we eat too much salt and we eat too much sugar. The simple advice is therefore:

- Eat more starchy foods such as potatoes, bread, rice and pasta.
- Eat more fruit and vegetables, whether fresh, frozen or tinned.
- When you eat dairy produce, choose the low-fat varieties.
- Eat lean meat, poultry and fish.

To these four basic food groups, a couple of extra pieces of advice should be added:

- Eat three meals a day. If you miss meals you are more likely to have fatty or sugary snacks to fill the gap – a bag of crisps or a chocolate bar.
- Drink water during the day.

We know we all need to eat less fat, and in particular less saturated/animal fat. Fat makes you fat and saturated fat increases your cholesterol level, both of which are risk factors for coronary heart disease. Yes, we all need to consume less sugar – whether it is sugar in tea and on cereals, or hidden in bought cakes, biscuits and sweets. We all need to eat less salt, whether you sprinkle it directly on to your meals, add it to cooking water or eat it hidden in bought snacks and other bought foods. But these all say 'Don't'. What is being said here is 'Do'.

- *Do* enjoy your food.
- *Do* eat a variety of different foods. Do you have chips with everything? Try some pasta meals. Try some rice meals. Try potatoes in another form.
- *Do* eat plenty of foods high in starch and fibre – potatoes, pasta, rice, lentils, beans. And do try to eat them without a huge smothering of butter or cheese or oil – try smaller amounts of low-fat alternatives or other sauces.
- *Do* eat lots of fruit and vegetables, both with your main meals and, if necessary, as snacks between meals. You cannot eat too much of them – and the more you eat, the less you are likely to eat fatty foods.
- *Do* try and cut down on fat. Use low-fat alternatives – spreads, yoghurt, cheeses. Use more bread, less spread. Buy skimmed or semi-skimmed milk. And remember that fat is often hidden in burgers, sausages, pies and salamis, so buy them less frequently.
- *Do* try and eat less sugary foods such as bought biscuits and cakes and snack bars. Eat more fruit instead.

Conclusion

Later in the book you will find specific chapters that give much more detail on how you can reduce the risk of suffering from heart disease and improving your chances of recovery after a heart attack:

- Chapter 8 looks in detail at how you can give up smoking and how you can develop strategies that will help you.
- Chapter 7 gives a detailed breakdown of exercise routines that can be adopted after a heart attack and what you need to do once you have recovered from a heart attack. It is the latter section that is most important if you are trying to reduce your risk of heart diesease.
- You will find more detailed advice on food in Chapter 10 towards the end of the book.

4 Consequences of a heart attack

In this chapter we will look at some of the practical results of a heart attack – what it feels like, what treatment you will be given, what tests might be administered to you, how a heart attack might affect you psychologically and what you might be offered in the way of surgery.

Physical impact

When we talk about a heart attack it is invariably the physical symptoms that loom largest in the conversation, simply because for most people who go through a heart attack it is the most painful, uncomfortable and frightening experience they have ever had. (This is not to say that all heart attacks are the same. Indeed, some people have what are known as 'silent' heart attacks – they do not realise that a heart attack has occurred, life goes on as normal and it is not until subsequent tests are carried out that some damage to the heart muscle is detected, indicating an earlier heart attack.) This opening section will therefore look at the various symptoms that may occur. It is as well to remember, however, that few heart attack patients suffer from all the symptoms; for example, although pain can be acute, in some cases the heart attack gives rise to no or very little pain.

It is very important that as many people in the general population are aware of what the symptoms of a heart attack are, so that they can act swiftly to alert the health services – both ambulance *and* GP. One of the best ways of ensuring survival of a heart attack patient is to get them into hospital as quickly as possible. This is a point that will be returned to later in the book.

Pain

The most familiar sensation associated with a heart attack is pain. If you have already suffered from angina, then you will have some familiarity with the level of pain and the parts of the body involved. It usually starts in the centre of the chest and spreads out to take in one or both arms, especially the left arm. It can spread to the neck and up into the chin. It may come on very quickly or increase in intensity quite slowly – perhaps over an hour or so. Or it may come and go intermittently. As it gets more severe it is usually described as the worst pain ever experienced – 'overwhelming', 'crushing', 'constricting', 'breathtaking' are typical adjectives.

Nausea and indigestion

After pain, perhaps the most common symptom is that of indigestion and feeling sick. In many cases breathlessness, 'feeling a bit queer' and indigestion are the early signs of a heart attack, and time is wasted taking anti-indigestion pills instead of contacting the GP and the ambulance. Ninety per cent of heart attack patients describe indigestion as one of their symptoms; furthermore, they truly believe they have acute indigestion, even though they may have never had it before and it may not be associated with eating anything abnormal or a heavy meal.

'Oh it's nothing, dear, just a bit of indigestion, I must have overdone it with that big meal last night,' is sometimes the last thing that a heart attack patient is heard to say.

Breathlessness

Associated with the pain is usually breathlessness. This is partly due to the pain itself and partly due to the damaged heart failing in its task of getting sufficient oxygen around the body.

The breathlessness will in turn lead to weakness and an overwhelming need for rest. Perhaps the symptoms come on while you are out for a walk, in which case all you will want to do is sit down somewhere – anywhere – and not move. You feel as if you are gasping for life and have no desire to move.

Other symptoms

If you have a heart attack you might faint. You will undoubtedly look pale, grey or even bluish around the face and may complain of feeling sweaty or clammy. You might feel cold and clammy. Because of the discomfort in the arm or neck, you might be moving your arms or head around to try and get them comfortable. You may feel a tingling in the fingers, especially in the ring and little fingers.

A heart attack may give rise to what are known as *cardiac arrhythmias*. An arrhythmia means that something that normally works rhythmically goes out of rhythm, i.e. it goes haywire. The heart normally beats rhythmically, but a heart attack can throw it completely out of its regular rhythm and this can add a very serious complication to what is already a serious problem. Cardiac arrhythmias most commonly occur in the first four hours after a heart attack. Ambulance crews usually have equipment on hand to correct them, which is one of the reasons for getting an ambulance to a heart attack patient as quickly as possible.

Psychological impact

Many people are aware of the physical symptoms of a heart attack and may have some idea of the process of recovery – the rush to hospital, the two or three days in a coronary care unit (CCU), the move to a general ward as they get better, the return to home and the gradual recovery of a normal life. What is not always so readily realised is that these stages are accompanied by a process of psychological adjustment that at times can be as alarming as the physical side of a heart attack.

This section looks at these psychological stages in broad terms, to give you some insight into what might be going on in your own head or in the head of someone you love during and after a heart attack. You must understand that these stages are not a strict and rigid sequence. Anxiety can arise at many stages; a sense of loss might not appear until well after the heart attack patient has gone home, as the realisation gradually dawns that they might not be able to return to their old job; denial can occur at any stage, from the onset of symptoms to long after the event.

Anxiety
Anxiety is associated with uncertainty and is perhaps the most overwhelming emotion that afflicts you when you suffer a heart attack:

- It starts with the initial symptoms – 'Oh my God, what's happening to me?'
- It gets worse as a doctor and an ambulance appear and whisk you off to hospital.
- After all sorts of needles are stuck into you and you rather lose track of things, you end up in a CCU, surrounded by machines (many of which are hooked up to your body) and busy people. 'What are they doing to me?'
- Then just as you get used to the security of the CCU, you are moved to a general ward. 'What happens if I have another heart attack,

away from all those life-saving machines?'

- Then – even worse – you are packed off home, terrified of doing anything that might bring on another heart attack. Everything – climbing stairs, going outside, even cleaning your teeth too vigorously – fills you with fear and trepidation.

All these situations, and many more in the days and months after a heart attack, can give rise to a sense of anxiety. And it must be remembered that anxiety can afflict not just the heart attack patient but also their family – indeed, at times the family may be more anxious than the patient. This anxiety can be increased if you do not know what is happening or what is being done to you. It is therefore important that as much as possible is explained to you; this may require some firm questioning by you or your family, and some thorough reading around the subject. This book will help a lot in giving you a clear understanding of all that is happening to you.

Gradually, as you adjust to the various situations you find yourself in and you gain a clearer insight into what comes next in the recovery process, your sense of anxiety will diminish. This is part of the process of adjustment.

Fear
Where anxiety stops and fear starts is often difficult to define. Anxiety, as we have seen, has more to do with uncertainty, while fear concerns the possibility of something specific (and unpleasant) occurring.

- To begin with it is fear of dying.
- Then there is the fear of another heart attack.
- There is fear of being a permanent invalid.
- There is fear of not being able to work again or of losing one's job or of having to take a drop in salary, with all the attendant implications on family finances.

Many of these fears will be unfounded and can be dispelled by clear information from the hospital staff or GP. Those fears that are real can be addressed once you have the correct information and in many cases medical staff or staff from other agencies can help resolve them satisfactorily. The important point is that you must be prepared to discuss your fears with the relevant staff, and when you don't understand something, say so and ask for a clearer explanation.

Loss

There will undoubtedly be a sense of loss at some stage during the recovery process. It may be the loss of what was assumed to be a healthy heart. It may be the sense of loss of what was assumed to be a healthy lifestyle, or of a lifestyle that you had got used to or felt comfortable with, or of a sense of your self-worth.

If it is necessary to change jobs or take early retirement because of the heart attack, there may be a profound sense of loss at the disappearance of the job. For many people their job is their life, their description – 'What are you?' 'Oh, I'm a train driver/fireman/doctor.' How do you answer that question if you are forced to give up being a train driver or fireman or doctor?

Depression

Anxiety, fear and loss can all give rise to depression. Depression in this case is not merely a question of feeling a bit low: it can be crushing and all-pervasive. If you are not prepared for it you can confuse it with the physical symptoms that you are also suffering.

You will feel drained by depression. You will not want to do anything. You will constantly feel close to tears or find yourself crying for no apparent reason. For a while life may feel such an effort that it has no point. This can be distressing even if you have been forewarned about it; if it comes as a complete surprise, it can be very upsetting and can interfere with the expected pattern of recovery.

It is important to understand that depression is a normal part of the process of adjustment to and recovery from any serious event or disease, not just a heart attack. While it lasts it can feel awful, but you must understand that it will pass. For some people it lasts a few days, for others it can last longer, and it may return to varying degrees at certain points in the recovery process. It is a part of the process of coming to terms with what has happened A heart attack is a life-threatening event, it is frightening, it can cause loss of self-image or of self-worth, and such loss and fear give rise to grief and depression.

Denial

Some people cope with the trauma of a heart attack by a process of denial. For example, they deny that they are experiencing the symptoms of a heart attack – 'No, it's just indigestion, leave me alone and I'll be all right.' (Interestingly, those who have already had a previous heart attack and cardiologists – both groups of people who should know better – are famous for ignoring the symptoms of a heart attack.)

Denial can manifest itself in the assertion, while still in hospital, that 'I am not at all worried by what has happened.' This is obvious nonsense. While a heart attack can be survived, it is a serious event and is not to be taken lightly.

Some heart attack patients express scepticism about whether they have had a heart attack and may even go so far as flatly to contradict the diagnosis. An even more extreme example of denial is when the heart attack patient 'tempts fate' by indulging in inappropriate behaviour – manically trying to do the garden as soon as they get home, going on massive drinking binges, driving the car with reckless abandon. This may not harm them, but invariably causes huge distress to other members of their family, particularly their partners.

Denial may be a short-term method of coping, particularly in a well-informed individual. It becomes a serious problem when it interferes with or is used to block medical treatment and subsequent rehabilitation.

Medicines

A heart attack patient can be treated with a number of medicines or drugs, from the time immediately after the heart attack, when crisis management is the order of the day, to long-term drug treatment to stabilise the symptoms of heart disease and reduce the risk of subsequent heart attacks.

Analgesia (pain relief) and thrombolytics (clot-busting drugs) are administered as soon after a heart attack as is possible. Then beta-blockers, vasodilators, anticoagulants, antiarrhythmics, diuretics and cholesterol-controlling drugs are used as part of the long-term management of coronary heart disease to prevent subsequent heart attacks and to control some of the symptoms of coronary heart disease.

Pain relief
As has already been explained, one of the most significant symptoms of a heart attack is pain – in the chest, in the arms, in the neck, in the chin. It can be completely crushing and overpowering. Once a doctor or paramedic has appeared on the scene, one of the priorities is to administer pain relief to the heart attack patient. This pain relief always involves injections of opium-based drugs as these are the strongest and most effective painkillers we have. In the UK diamorphine (heroin) is

most commonly used; in other countries morphine is used.

Not only do the opiate drugs give rapid and effective pain relief, but they also reduce the state of anxiety that the patient is undoubtedly suffering and thus allow them to relax.

Clot-busters

As has already been explained, a heart attack is usually caused by one of the furred-up deposits (and often it is only a small one) in the arteries serving the heart having a clot forming on top of it and blocking the artery so that a section of heart muscle is starved of oxygen and nutrients. Alternatively, a clot detaches from the deposit and blocks the blood vessel elsewhere around the heart. If a drug can be administered that dissolves the clots blocking or limiting blood circulation in the arteries, the blood circulation can be opened up and the muscle damage limited.

Such drugs now exist. Known colloquially as 'clot-busters', their technical name is *thrombolytics* – a *thrombus* is a clot and a *lytic agent* is something that breaks down or removes something. Streptokinase is the most commonly used clot-buster or thrombolytic, but alteplase is another similar drug that might be used. They have to be administered slowly, so are run into the body via a drip into one of the veins, usually in the arm.

Thrombolytic drugs cannot be used for every heart attack patient; if the patient is already liable to bleed, for example from recent surgery or from a stomach ulcer, then clot-busters are not a good idea. However, for most heart attack patients it is important to administer them as soon as possible. It is for this reason that the emergency services need to be activated as soon as a heart attack is suspected – phone the ambulance service and then the GP, telling both that a suspected heart attack is occurring or has occurred. As soon as the GP is there the pain relief can be administered; and the sooner the patient is got into hospital the sooner the thrombolytic drug can be administered and the risk of subsequent heart attacks reduced.

Aspirin also has blood-thinning and clot-dissolving capabilities, and is now routinely administered as soon as possible after a heart attack. It then becomes one of the drugs that heart attack patients take regularly for the rest of their lives.

Beta blockers

Beta blockers are a group of drugs that limit the increase in heart rate (the number of times the heart beats per minute) and blood pressure that occur during exercise and during periods of emotion such as anger or anxiety. Specifically they reduce the effect of the hormone adrenaline. They are used not only in the long-term management of heart attack patients, but also for the treatment of angina.

Drugs can be referred to by their trade name (beginning with a capital letter) or by their chemical name (beginning with a small letter). For example, the most commonly prescribed beta blockers are:

- Tenormin/atenolol
- Inderal/propranolol
- Lopressor and Betaloc/metoprolol
- Trasicor/oxprenolol

All drugs have side-effects, some more serious than others. Beta blockers can cause:

- Tiredness.
- Cold extremities, e.g. fingers and toes.
- Rashes.
- Sleep disturbances and nightmares.
- Sickness and stomach upset.
- Difficulty obtaining erection or maintaining an erection during sexual intercourse.

If you have any of these side-effects, tell your doctor and ask if you can try a different variety of beta blocker – there are a number of types and one may agree with you better than another.

Nitrates

Nitrates are vasodilators and vasodilators, very simply, widen the arteries – *vaso* refers to the blood vessels and *to dilate* means to widen. They can have three major effects:

- By widening the arteries they can reduce the effect of the furring-up of the coronary arteries.
- They can help to lower blood pressure.
- They can reduce the amount of work the heart has to do.

Nitrates are used in the treatment of angina – the pain in the chest that occurs when the heart is asked to do more work than the furred-up coronary arteries can cope with. Angina can affect people who have not had a heart attack as well as those who have suffered from a heart attack in the past. The idea is that when an angina attack comes on or when one is anticipated, e.g. when a period of activity, exercise or love-making is planned, the nitrate pill is placed under the tongue or between the gum and upper lip, or chewed, or a nitrate spray is used. Nitrates act very fast, either removing the chest pain or preventing it coming on.

The most commonly prescribed nitrates are:

- GTN/glyceryl trinitrate
- Isordil and Sorbitrate/isosorbide dinitrate
- Ismo 20 or Monit/isosorbide mononitrate

Nitrates can also cause a number of side-effects:

- A throbbing headache.
- Dizziness – take the nitrates sitting down until you get used to them.
- A rash.
- Hot flushes.

As with other drugs, talk to your doctor if you get any of these side-effects and find out if any of the other nitrates suit you better.

Other vasodilators
There are various other vasodilators used in the long-term management of heart attack patients. They include, among others:

- ACE inhibitors.
- Calcium antagonists.
- Alpha-1 antagonists.

The important point to remember is that whatever they are called and whatever their precise means of action (and this is not the sort of book to go into the detailed action of all the drugs you might be prescribed), they all act to widen the blood vessels, in particular the coronary arteries, to bring down blood pressure and to reduce the work-load on the heart. Typical drugs in this group include:

- Adalat/nifedipine
- Cordilox/verapimil

- Tildiem/diltiazem
- Capoten or Acepril/captopril
- Innovace/enalapril
- Apresoline/hydralazine
- Hypovase/prazosin

There are a number of possible side-effects, depending on the specific drug prescribed. They include:

- Drowsiness.
- Fatigue.
- Changes in the sense of taste.
- Persistent dry cough.
- A rash.
- Hot flushes.
- Headache.

As with other drugs, if you are bothered by any of these side-effects, discuss the situation with your GP and ask if other similar drugs could be tried that might be more suited to you.

Anticoagulants

Anticoagulants all reduce the risk of blood clots forming in the arteries and causing a subsequent blockage. However, they also reduce the risk of blood clots forming elsewhere, so the more powerful anticoagulants have to be monitored very carefully; if you are on any of these strong anticoagulants your doctor will check your blood regularly.

The most commonly used anticoagulant is aspirin and this is now routinely prescribed for everyone who has had a heart attack, unless they also have stomach ulcers. If you have had a heart attack and are put on a daily dose of aspirin, it is not for pain relief but to reduce the risk of blood clots forming in the blood system. The use of more powerful anticoagulants is far less common; they were prescribed for other problems with the heart – for example, after coronary artery bypass surgery or if there are problems with the heart valves – but even these are rare nowadays.

The most powerful of the anticoagulants is called warfarin. If you are on warfarin you will have regular blood checks to see that the prescribed dose is at the right level – if it is too high there is a risk of uncontrolled bleeding. You should be issued with a blue warfarin card and you should tell any doctor, dentist, hospital or chemist that you are on the drug. Aspirin can increase the effect of warfarin and is sometimes combined with warfarin for anticoagulant treatment, but this is always under very careful medical supervision. Aspirin (even aspirin in a cold relief compound) normally should never be taken if you are on warfarin treatment, unless prescribed by your doctor.

The various anticoagulant drugs have the following names:

- Angettes or Caprin or Nu-seals/aspirin
- Marevan/warfarin

Antiarrhythmics

The antiarrhythmic drugs are used to keep the heart beating regularly – often after a heart attack it doesn't beat as regularly as it used to. Some of the antiarrhythmic drugs also make the heart beat stronger.

The most commonly used drugs in this group are:

- Lanoxin/digoxin
- Cordilox or Securon/verapamil
- Cordarone X/amiodarone
- Dirythmin SA or Isomide or Rythmodan/disopyramide (not used a lot now)
- Mexitil/mexiletene (not used a lot now)

As with other drugs, there are some potential side-effects. These can include sickness and loss of appetite.

Diuretics

Diuretics are commonly known as 'water pills'. This is because they act to remove excess water from the body. If the heart is not working efficiently, water can accumulate in the body, causing swollen ankles and breathlessness. Diuretics act to remove this surplus water via the kidneys. As a result, the heart has less work to do.

Diuretics work by removing sodium from the body and the water goes with the sodium. Sodium is most commonly found in salt, so if you are on diuretics you should not eat excess salt or salty foods, otherwise you will counteract the effect of the diuretics.

The most commonly used diuretics are:

- Burinex or Burinex K/bumetanide

- Frumil or Frusene or Lasikal or Lasilactone or Lasix or Lasix + K or Lasoride/frusemide

Again, there are a number of side-effects. Going to the toilet more frequently is the most obvious one. You may also get muscle cramps or muscle weakness; this is often caused by a lack of potassium, and can be counteracted by eating plenty of fresh fruit and vegetables, particularly bananas, oranges and tomatoes. If your doctor thinks that potassium loss is a problem for you, they can prescribe water pills with extra potassium in them – the drug name usually has a K after it. Some men on water pills may have problems with getting an erection.

Cholesterol-lowering drugs

If you have a high blood cholesterol level, there is an increased risk of furring-up of the arteries continuing. Many people lower their cholesterol levels by taking more exercise and changing their diet, but some people have high cholesterol levels that are resistant to such changes. If you fall into this latter category and you have had a heart attack you are likely to be put on one of the cholesterol-lowering drugs. It is important to realise that such drugs will be most effective when they are taken as part of an overall cholesterol-lowering programme, including more exercise and dietary changes; they are not a substitute for lifestyle changes.

There are various categories of such drugs. The most commonly prescribed are:

- Lipantil/fenofibrate.
- Lopid/gemfibrozil.
- Modalim/ciprofibrate.
- Questran/cholestyramine.
- Colestid/colestipol.
- Zocor/simvastatin.
- Lipostat/pravastatin.
- Lescol/fluvastatin.

There are various side-effects depending on the category of drug used, but the most common are upsets to the digestive tract – wind, diarrhoea and occasionally sickness – while the most serious is muscle cramp or myositis.

Tests

After a heart attack you will be given a number of tests, some shortly after the incident, to make sure that a heart attack has occurred and to establish its severity, and some later on, to help the doctors decide whether or not you need surgery or further investigations.

Blood tests

When you go into hospital you inevitably undergo various blood tests – a sample of blood is taken from a vein in your arm and various tests are then carried out on it.

After a heart attack there is a very important blood test that is always carried out. Heart muscle cells contain various enzymes – chemicals – that are not found elsewhere in the body. During a heart attack, however slight, some heart muscle cells will be damaged and these enzymes will be released into the bloodstream. Blood tests to monitor the levels of these enzymes released into the blood stream will help to determine whether a heart attack has occurred and how severe it has been.

You will also have cholesterol tests, not only while you are in hospital but also as a regular feature of your visits to your GP and cardiac clinic. There are two sorts of cholesterol test. The first uses a pin-prick sample of blood and gives the total cholesterol level in a few minutes. A more detailed picture is often required, though, and to obtain this a sample of blood is drawn from a vein in your arm and sent off to the laboratory for analysis; the result will take a day or so to come back.

ECG

ECG is short for *electrocardiogram*; it is a printout of the electrical activity within the heart.

The human body drives its muscles by means of tiny electrical impulses. The heart muscle is no different and needs its regular electrical impulses to function. These impulses to the heart muscle have a normal pattern; after a heart attack they show a degree of abnormality that will give the doctors a fair idea of what areas of heart muscle have been damaged.

To take an ECG electrical conductors (electrodes) are attached to the wrists and legs and other electrodes are attached to the chest. Wires from these electrodes are connected to a recorder and when it is switched on it detects and magnifies the tiny electrical impulses from the heart and prints them out as a continuous tracing on paper. If you look at this printout you will see that it has various spikes and dips.

Characteristic changes in this pattern indicate what sort of damage the heart has suffered and whether it was recent or some time in the past.

If you have suffered a heart attack you will soon become used to having an ECG taken. It is a relatively easy test to run and interpret, so not only do hospitals make use of them, but also many health centres are geared up to taking and interpreting them.

In some cases you might be wired up to a small portable ECG recorder for 24 hours. The recorder is about the size of a personal stereo and clips on to the belt. You are then sent home and asked to carry out your normal activities, keeping a diary of what you are doing. When you hand the equipment back in to hospital the staff correlate your diary times with the heart trace and look for any abnormalities that might occur during particular activities.

Exercise ECG

An ECG taken when you are at rest will give the doctors a lot of information. However, at some time or other after you have had a heart attack you will have an exercise ECG taken. This is simply what it says it is – an ECG taken while you are exercising.

The exercise is either on a treadmill or an exercise bike. You are connected to the electrodes of an ECG recorder and then asked to exercise until your heart rate has reached a certain level, or you have reached a stage where you are puffed out and weary, or you are suffering from chest pains, or the ECG indicates significant changes. The exercise is intended to be hard work, but it is not exhausting; the first time you are likely to come up against an exercise ECG is a few days after you have gone into hospital with a heart attack and it may come as a pleasant surprise to discover quite how much you can manage.

An exercise ECG gives a lot more information about the heart than a resting ECG, particularly how well the heart is able to cope with work. It also gives valuable information as to what sort of future treatment, e.g. surgery, might be necessary.

Echocardiography

You are probably aware of the way that bats detect surrounding objects by emitting very high-pitched squeaks and listening for the echoes. Sonar uses a similar system to map the seabed, bouncing sound waves off undersea hills and valleys. And anyone who has had a baby will have had an ultrasound scan to produce a picture of the baby in the womb.

A similar ultrasound system can be used to take pictures of the heart. This is known as *echocardiography*. An ultrasound probe is placed on the chest and the chest smeared with a jelly to establish a better contact. The probe is moved around to build up a picture of the heart and, in some cases, an idea of the flow of blood through the heart. It is a completely painless and non-invasive procedure for the patient, but it is not simple and the resulting images need careful interpretation by the doctor.

Echocardiography is not used as a routine test if you have had a heart attack. However, if there is a suspicion that the valves in your heart are diseased, then it is much more likely to be used. It also gives information about the extent of the muscle damage to the heart.

Angiogram

An angiogram is carried out when the doctors want to see precisely how diseased the blood vessels of the heart have become or to get a detailed idea of the functioning of the heart itself. It is therefore used for angina patients as well as for people who have suffered a heart attack. It is a complex procedure, carried out in the cardiac department of the hospital. It may be carried out while you are already in hospital, for example after a heart attack, or you may be asked to come in as a day-case or short-stay patient.

What happens is very simple to explain, but takes time to carry out. A fine flexible tube is inserted into a blood artery in your groin or arm. Local anaesthetic is used to ensure that this is relatively painless. The tube is then manoeuvred through your blood system until it reaches your heart – you can see this being done on a TV monitor if you ask. This might sound rather alarming, but it causes no discomfort. Furthermore you will be on an ECG monitor so that the staff can tell if any problems are developing.

Once the tip of the tube is in the right place a fluid is injected down the tube. This fluid shows up on X-rays (it is called *radio-opaque*, i.e. it blocks X-rays), and allows the cardiologist to take a series of X-ray pictures of the heart and the coronary arteries. The tip of the tube is also able to measure blood pressure, so a detailed picture of the functioning of the heart can be built up.

If the insertion is to be in your groin, you may be asked to shave the area – if you are nervous of doing this yourself a member of hospital staff should be able to do it for you. You will be fasted for a few hours before the test; this reduces any risk of your feeling sick during it. You may be given an injection or a pill to relax you. During the test you may be aware of some strange sensations when they run the radio-opaque fluid through the tube; it may be a hot flushing feeling and you may feel as if you've wet yourself (although you haven't). After the test you will have a few stitches in the arm; if the groin has been used as an entry point, a 10–20 minute pressure is usually enough to close the hole, although you will have to rest with your leg straight for another few hours before you can get up. You may feel a bit weak for a while and if you are in on a day-case basis you will have to get someone else to drive you home.

There are slight risks attached to this test; bruising often occurs around the site of insertion of the tube. Very, very rarely the test can bring on a heart attack; the investigation will therefore only be carried out if your doctor feels that the benefits of the information gained far outweigh the very slight risk involved. If you are in any way concerned about the risks, discuss the situation with your doctor, who should explain things in more detail than is possible here.

Surgery

When the average layman hears of heart surgery he tends to think of heart transplants. In fact heart transplants comprise only a tiny proportion of operations to treat heart disease and the heart disease usually has to be very severe before a heart transplant is considered.

In this section we will look at the more common surgical procedures carried out to treat coronary heart disease. Strictly speaking, coronary angioplasty and the insertion of stents are not surgical procedures, but they have been grouped here as they both require a short stay in hospital (assuming the patient isn't already in hospital).

Angioplasty

Coronary angioplasty is in some ways similar to carrying out a cardiac catheterisation in that both techniques require the insertion of a fine tube into the blood system, either through the groin or the arm. However, this tube is much finer than for an angiogram as it is designed to go into much smaller blood vessels – the coronary arteries.

The coronary arteries, as already mentioned, encircle the heart like a crown. They supply the heart muscle with oxygen and nutrients, without which the heart cannot function. As we have seen, in coronary heart disease these arteries become furred up, and not enough oxygen and nutrients can get to the heart muscle. This causes angina, and if part of the deposits that fur up these arteries goes on to block a coronary artery you have a heart attack. The aim of angioplasty is to open up the areas of blockage or furring up in the coronary arteries, thus reducing the symptoms of angina and the risk of a heart attack.

Once the guiding tube is positioned at the start of the relevant coronary artery, a thin guide-wire is passed beyond the narrowed segment and a thin catheter with a small sausage-shaped balloon near the end is then passed over or along the wire and inflated in the area where the artery is narrowed. This opens up the narrowing, squashing the furred-up deposits to the sides of the artery wall. The balloon remains inflated for a few minutes, then is deflated and removed, leaving the artery no longer narrowed. Blood flow to the heart muscle is improved, the symptoms of angina should be removed and the risk of a subsequent heart attack diminished. The balloon is much less than ¼ of an inch – only 2 or 3 millimetres in width – so you don't have to worry about some party balloon bursting out of your chest.

Angioplasty is not a technique that is suitable for all coronary heart disease patients. If the area of narrowing in the coronary arteries is too inaccessible, or if there are too many areas of narrowing or they are too long, then angioplasty is not for you. And if you do undergo angioplasty there is a small risk that, during the procedure, it will completely block the coronary artery rather than open it up; this poses a serious risk to the heart and if it happens you may have to have an immediate coronary artery bypass operation. The chances of this are low, but it will always be explained to you before angioplasty that there is a risk that it will lead to you having to have an urgent operation.

In most cases – 60 to 70 per cent – the technique is very successful, though. Furthermore it has many advantages – a short hospital stay of a few days, the avoidance of major surgery and the ease with which it can be repeated if necessary.

Stents

The use of stents is a relatively new technique. It is a development of angioplasty, whereby the narrowing of the coronary artery is expanded by the inflation of a balloon and then held open permanently by a tiny wire-mesh tube that remains inside the artery after the balloon has been deflated and removed.

As far as the patient is concerned, the practicalities of the procedure are the same. A tube is inserted into a blood vessel in the arm or groin

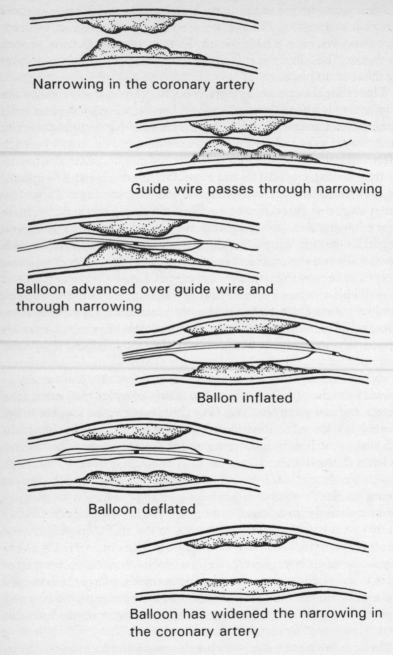

Narrowing in the coronary artery

Guide wire passes through narrowing

Balloon advanced over guide wire and through narrowing

Ballon inflated

Balloon deflated

Balloon has widened the narrowing in the coronary artery

Fig. 7 *Coronary angioplasty.*

and then manoeuvred until the tip of the tube is in the narrowed area of the coronary artery. The balloon carrying the stent is then inflated, stretching the wire-mesh tube out so that it opens out the area of narrowing. The balloon is then deflated and the tube withdrawn, leaving the stent in place.

This is not the end of the story, though. A piece of wire-mesh tube in an artery is a foreign body and the body tends to deal with it by forming a clot around it. If this were allowed to happen the coronary artery would very rapidly be blocked again and you would be back where you started. To prevent the formation of clots on the stent, various treatments are available; you might be put on a course of warfarin, the strongest of the anticoagulants or anti-clotting drugs. As we saw earlier in this chapter, if you are on warfarin you will have to have regular blood checks to ensure that the warfarin is at the right level. After three months the cells of the artery wall will have grown around the wire mesh of the stent and there is no longer the risk of clots forming on it. The warfarin will then be stopped. However warfarin is used only in this procedure for high risks of angioplasty. Alternatively, you could be put on a combination of aspirin and heparin (another anticoagulant). Stents are now being produced that are pre-coated with heparin, thus reducing the need for anticoagulant drugs after they have been inserted.

As with angioplasty, the insertion of a stent is relatively straightforward procedure for the patient, but quite a complex business for the doctors. Because it is a relatively new technique, it is not possible to say whether it offers benefits over ordinary angioplasty. However, it is a technique that is still developing and there are likely to be further advances in the future.

Bypass surgery

Coronary artery bypass surgery (or coronary artery bypass graft, CABG or cabbage, as it is more usually known as in the medical world) constitutes more than half the heart operations carried out in the UK. Very simply, this operation uses a piece of a blood vessel taken from elsewhere in the body to bypass the blocked or limited bits of the coronary arteries. This restores normal blood supply to the heart muscle, and removes the pain of angina in the great majority of cases and reduces the discomfort in the remainder.

It is a major operation. The breastbone is cut open from top to bottom and the chest cavity opened up, giving good access to the heart, which lies at the centre of the chest. A heart/lung bypass machine then takes over the role of the heart and lungs while the surgery is carried out on the heart. To create the bypasses for the blocked sections of coronary artery, spare arteries from inside the chest wall are usually used, although in many cases lengths of vein are taken from the leg as well; as the leg is very well supplied with blood vessels, this poses no problems for the subsequent health of the leg. The distal part of arterial bypasses are then stitched into place, while in the case of veins they are connected from the aorta, the main blood vessel leaving the heart, to points on the coronary arteries beyond the areas of blockage. The heart/lung machine is then withdrawn and the chest closed up.

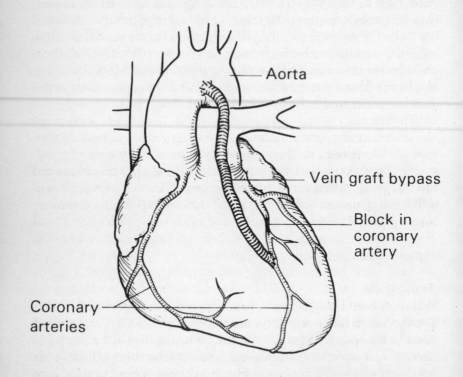

Fig. 8 *Coronary artery bypass surgery.*

Described like this, it may sound a complex operation. In fact it is a nowadays looked upon as a straightforward 're-plumbing' procedure and thousands of bypass operations are carried out in the UK each year. You will normally be in hospital for a couple of weeks – two or three days before the operation and about 6–8 days afterwards, first of all on an intensive care ward then on a general ward. If the veins are taken from the leg, you may have a coin-sized area of sensory loss due to unavoidable damage to the local sensory nerve. A depression syndrome may also occur on the first few postoperative days, but soon settles after that. The breast-bone will take anything up to three months to heal comfortably; during that time you may suffer quite a lot of pain, both in the chest and in the muscles of the neck, back and arms. Don't be afraid of using adequate and satisfactory pain relief for this discomfort; if you can relieve the pain you will be more relaxed and better able to heal yourself. There is no benefit whatsoever in stoically enduring pain, and no risk of somehow becoming 'addicted' to pain relief. You will also experience some pain and discomfort in the leg if this is where the bypass veins have been removed, as well as perhaps some swelling; the latter will be helped by wearing a support stocking and keeping the leg raised up on a stool whenever you sit down, particularly in the first few weeks, and raising up the foot end of your bed.

The relatively recent development in CABG operations – the use of the internal chest artery to create the bypass grafts – appears to give very good long-term results, particularly in younger patients.

Nearly 20,000 people a year in the UK have CABG operations and after 10 years it is expected that 60 per cent of the leg-vein grafts will still be working successfully and nearly 100 per cent of the mammary artery grafts. The result of the operation is improved if the blood cholesterol level can subsequently be kept low – this greatly reduces the risk of the new plumbing furring up.

Transplants

Although heart transplants can have a lot of publicity and media interest, they are in fact a very uncommon operation. They are only carried out at a few specialised centres in the UK and will only be offered to those people with serious advanced heart disease, who will probably have various other problems in addition to having suffered one or more heart attacks.

As with coronary artery bypass surgery, the chest has to be opened up and the patient switched over to an artificial heart/lung machine.

There the similarity ends, though, for the whole of the diseased heart (and sometimes the lungs) is removed and replaced with a healthy heart from a suitable donor. This is obviously a major surgical procedure and takes quite a few hours to complete.

In the past there have been major problems of rejection. The new heart has been recognised as something 'foreign' by the recipient's body, and attacked and rejected by the immune system. While this problem still remains, it has been lessened enormously by the development of new drugs, so that heart transplants now offer a very effective treatment for those people with very serious heart disease.

The risk of recurrence

One of the biggest questions that looms in your mind after you have had a heart attack is 'What is the risk of it happening to me again?' It's a frightful experience and the fear of another heart attack can often dominate your life.

Once you have had a heart attack, the risk of having another one is greatest in the few hours immediately after the first; this is why it is so important to alert your GP and the ambulance as soon as possible, so that you can be rushed into hospital and given the thrombolytic clot-busting drugs that will minimise this immediate risk. There is an even greater risk of arrhythmias, when the electrical stimulation of the heart goes haywire and the heart stops beating properly. This can be dealt with not only in the hospital but also in the ambulance on the way to hospital.

Once you are on the road to recovery and return to normal home life, the situation very much depends on what you do with your life. The various treatments and drugs described earlier in this chapter, in general, help in the relief of symptoms; for example, they will remove or reduce the pain of angina, they will allow you to lead a more active, less breathless life. However, what they won't do, in general, is significantly reduce your risk of having another heart attack. Only if you address the fundamental reasons responsible for your coronary heart disease will your risk of further heart attacks be reduced. This is not difficult, but requires a conscious decision on your part:

- If you smoke, you must seriously consider giving it up.
- You must examine ways in which you can increase the amount of exercise you take on a daily basis.

- You must look carefully at what you eat and perhaps change the balance of the various foods you consume.
- If you are overweight, particularly if you have abdominal fatness, you must do something about bringing your weight down.

These will all tackle the underlying reasons why you have coronary heart disease and will help bring the problem under control.

The role of complementary medicine

If you have a heart attack, you obviously need emergency treatment from the health service and you have to understand that your subsequent treatment will be firmly based within the health service, as will be explained in the next couple of chapters. However, you might be curious as to what, if any, help complementary medicine can offer if you have heart disease, e.g. angina or raised blood pressure, or are recovering from a heart attack.

There are two great advantages to complementary medicine when compared to regular medicine – time, and the fact that all branches of complementary medicine seek to treat the whole person. In terms of time, it is usual for a complementary medical specialist to see you for up to an hour at a time – perhaps an hour for the first consultation and half an hour for subsequent visits. This is considerably longer than you can expect from most doctors within the health service, not because they want to be rid of you as quickly as possible but simply because of the sheer pressure of numbers of patients. With more time at their disposal, complementary medical specialists are able to discuss with you a much broader range of features of the medical problem and can give you the opportunity to bring matters to the fore that you might not be able to discuss elsewhere. Indeed, many complementary specialists would see themselves as acting as a sounding board for the patient's thoughts and feelings on their medical problem, and in some cases acting as a counsellor, providing a 'safe' area where the patient can talk things over. This very much ties in with the concept of treating the whole person – not just a specific part of a person's body, but the whole body and mind and life that that person leads. This is not to suggest that such forms of medicine should be used instead of treatment from the health service – they should be used to complement what you are receiving from your doctors.

There are many branches of complementary medicine, but the

suggestion here is that of the major branches, medical herbalism, homoeopathy, perhaps acupuncture, massage and aromatherapy would have the most to offer if you suffer from heart disease or have had a heart attack:

- Herbal medicine, very simply, uses plants to prevent, treat and cure diseases. It is a very old skill, dating back to the beginnings of mankind – all of the ancient cultures had sophisticated systems of herbal medicine.
- Homoeopathy, in contrast, developed in the last century. It takes drugs that produce symptoms in a healthy individual that are similar to those of a particular disease, then uses the same drug, much diluted, to treat that disease. It is available within the health service – there are six homoeopathic hospitals in the NHS – although most people go to homoeopaths who practise independently.
- Acupuncture is an ancient Chinese art, whereby the organs and systems of the body can be treated via specific points on the body surface – these points are stimulated using needles. It is particularly effective at treating pain.
- Massage can be used to help relaxation and to ease out tense or knotted muscles – it is surprising how much tension we carry in our arms, shoulders and back, and massage can help to identify these areas, loosen them up. This in turn helps the healing process – a relaxed body heals more rapidly than a tense body – and promotes flexibility and movement, which in turn have a favourable impact on exercise and activity.
- Aromatherapy uses oils extracted from plants. These are worked into the body and their effect depends on the oils used – different oils have different properties. Aromatherapy is often associated with massage, and for the heart attack patient can promote healing and relaxation and raise energy levels.

If you go to see a complementary medical specialist it is impossible to predict what treatment and/or drugs they will suggest for you. One of the benefits of complementary medicine is that treatment tends to be much more individualised than that available within the health service. Medical herbalism, however, does make use of plants that have been used to treat heart problems for millennia. For example:

- Limeflower helps prevent arteriosclerosis. It is also a relaxant and

can be of use in managing high blood pressure.
- Garlic has blood thinning properties similar to aspirin. It also stimulates the circulation.
- Hawthorn and yarrow are also circulatory stimulants, and both help to normalise blood pressure.

If you want to make use of complementary medicine but don't know who to turn to, there are national registration bodies for most branches and these will have lists of specialists practising near you. The Yellow Pages will yield a list of many such specialists – start with the section headed Therapists and work out from there – although this gives no idea of how good they are and whether or not they might be suited to you. It is often preferable to ask people in your district whom they would recommend – nowadays many GPs have a good idea of what is available and are often happy to suggest individual specialists. If you are going to a cardiac rehabilitation centre, they may well be able to suggest people. Another line of enquiry is to ask at your local health- or wholefood shop.

5 The first 10 days

A minor heart attack

In a way the phrase 'a minor heart attack' is a contradiction in terms. During a heart attack, as already described, the blood supply to a portion of the heart muscle is cut off and the section of heart muscle involved is damaged. This is serious. Some heart attacks only show up in a very minor way on an ECG, however, and may not be clearly detected on subsequent ECGs from then on. These are called *subendocardial infarcts* and only involve a small portion of the heart muscle. They are still a dangerous condition, for they may give rise to a further heart attack or arrhythmia at a later stage.

However, occasionally full heart attacks do occur that do not result in a stay in hospital and, for various reasons, may not even involve the intervention of a doctor. It cannot be emphasised strongly enough that this situation is very rare, and it is an extremely unsatisfactory one to be in. If there is the slightest suspicion of a heart attack it is imperative that the GP is contacted immediately, and if you have chest pain lasting longer than 15 minutes then contact the ambulance and the GP.

Silent heart attacks

A silent heart attack is a heart attack that causes barely any detectable symptoms; they are more common with diabetics. Maybe you feel as if you've got a bit of indigestion, or you feel a little tired, or maybe you don't notice anything at all. You don't take any time off, the day goes on as normal, you feel a little off colour for a few days and that's the end of it. That is, until you have a routine health check, with an ECG, or you go into hospital for surgery and an ECG is taken, and an abnormality shows up on the ECG trace that indicates that a minor heart attack has occurred at some time.

Obviously, if you are completely unaware of any symptoms of a heart attack, then there's nothing you can do about it. However, if you have the slightest suspicion that you might be suffering from a heart attack, contact your GP. It is better to get them to see you and to discover that it is in fact only indigestion, than to leave things alone – 'I don't want to bother them, they're always so busy' – and run the risk of a subsequent, more serious heart attack a bit later, or heart arrhythmias that can be just as serious.

Remember, you are most at risk of fatal arrhythmias or another heart attack within the first 24 hours following the onset of chest pain or other symptoms.

Ignoring the symptoms

A silent heart attack may pass by with relatively few symptoms, whereas the situation is very different when you or a member of your family suddenly suffer any of the classic symptoms listed below, all of which suggest that a much larger chunk of heart muscle is affected. You or your family should not ignore these symptoms.

Now, it is true that the general public are remarkably ignorant of exactly what the typical symptoms of a heart attack are and one of the aims of this book is to remove this ignorance by providing a clear list of typical symptoms. These symptoms have already been detailed in an earlier chapter, but here they are again:

- The same sort of pain as is experienced with angina – a tightness or band around the chest; a gripping pain in the chest; a feeling of oppression in the chest; pain in the arms, especially the left arm, that may run down to the wrist and hand; pain in the neck and chin. At its worst this pain can be the most severe ever experienced.
- A feeling of indigestion, often not associated with eating anything out of the ordinary like a large meal; the great majority of patients describe and truly believe they have indigestion.
- A feeling of uselessness in one or both arms.
- Tingling in the fingers, especially the ring and little fingers.
- Nausea and vomiting.
- Breathlessness.
- Exhaustion.
- Feeling clammy and sweaty.
- Looking pale, grey or even slightly bluish around the face.
- Feeling 'odd', 'peculiar', 'strange', 'dizzy'.

It is important to realise that these constitute a wide range of symptoms and you may only suffer a selection of them. If the chest pain is mild, there might be a temptation to explain away the other symptoms as indigestion, a tummy upset, something funny with your arm, feeling under the weather, or whatever, and to do nothing about it. People do just this – they ignore the symptoms. And if they have already had a heart attack before, they seem to be particularly prone to ignoring symptoms – maybe it's trying to pretend that they aren't going through the same thing again; maybe it's a disbelief that it could happen again.

Whatever the reason for doing it, you must understand that any delay in contacting the medical services is potentially suicidal. The risk of a subsequent heart attack is high, and the risk of a fatal arrhythmia (this is when the electrical stimulation of the heart goes haywire, to the extent that it kills you) is very high.

It is far better to call out the doctor and ambulance and then to find that, although you are ill, it has not been a heart attack, than to delay calling them out – 'I'll go and see the doctor tomorrow if I'm still feeling lousy' – because if you leave things that long you may be dead by the time they do see you.

A heart attack – what happens

A heart attack will send you into the coronary care unit (CCU) of your nearest district hospital. You will stay in hospital for five to seven days if you have no further complications, longer if there are complications, and will then be sent home to continue the process of recovery and rehabilitation.

The period after a heart attack is normally divided into four phases:

phase 1 The period spent in hospital (weeks 1–2).

phase 2 The first 6 weeks spent at home (weeks 3–9).

phase 3 The subsequent 6–12 weeks, when you should be on a cardiac rehabilitation programme that involves exercise, advice and relaxation (weeks 1 to 16 or 22).

phase 4 The rest of your life after the cardiac rehabilitation programme has finished, when you should be putting into action and profiting from the advice you have received in phases 1, 2 and 3.

This chapter is looking at phase 1, your entry into hospital and subsequent stay there.

The first hours

This section is largely addressed to the person who has to look after a heart attack patient when the heart attack strikes. It gives essential advice on the course of action to be followed to get the patient into hospital and undergoing treatment as fast as possible. If you have already had a heart attack, or you suffer from the symptoms of coronary heart disease and are at high risk of a heart attack, all members of your family, your friends and people you work with should be aware of this advice. It might save your life.

The symptoms

A heart attack can strike at any time of the day or night, anywhere – at home, at work, on a walk, on a boat, on a plane, anywhere at all. The symptoms might come on very suddenly or they might come on gradually. You might wake up with them and be aware of them gradually getting worse or they might leave you pole-axed on the golf course in the middle of a game.

The essential feature is that you, or most likely someone with you, responds to these symptoms immediately. At the risk of becoming tedious, these symptoms are:

- The same sort of pain as is experienced with angina – a tightness or band around the chest; a gripping pain in the chest; a feeling of oppression in the chest; pain in the arms, especially the left arm, that may run down to the wrist and hand; pain in the neck and chin. At its worst this pain can be the most severe ever experienced.
- A feeling of indigestion, often not associated with eating anything out of the ordinary like a large meal.
- A feeling of uselessness in one or both arms.
- Tingling in the fingers, especially the ring and little fingers.
- Nausea and vomiting.
- Breathlessness.
- Exhaustion.
- Feeling clammy and sweaty.
- Looking pale, grey or even slightly bluish around the face.
- Feeling 'odd', 'peculiar', 'strange', 'dizzy'.

There are great variations in these symptoms, and in old people there may be no pain, merely weakness, collapse and breathlessness.

Calling the emergency services

After a heart attack there is a great risk of further heart attacks and serious arrhythmias known as *ventricular fibrillation* – both can be fatal, i.e. they can kill you. They can be dealt with or prevented if you are already in an ambulance or in hospital, which is why it is essential that any heart attack symptoms are responded to as soon as possible. Because of ignorance of heart attack symptoms and therefore delays in contacting the medical services, 25 per cent of heart attack patients do not survive the first hour after a heart attack and 50 per cent do not reach hospital alive. The faster you can get a doctor and ambulance to the heart attack patient, the greater chance they have of getting rapid treatment and of not becoming one of these grim statistics.

The following course of action is therefore recommended.

- Phone 999 for an ambulance. You are perfectly entitled to do this – it is not something that only doctors can do. When you phone 999 you will be asked which emergency service you need. Say 'Ambulance.' You will be transferred to the ambulance control desk and asked a series of questions about who the patient is, where the patient is and what the problem is. The answer to the last question is 'Suspected heart attack.' You also need to give a clear address. Above all, do not panic – answer the questions as they are asked and do not try to blurt out information out of sequence.
- Then phone the patient's health centre or clinic or surgery. Ask to speak to their GP as a matter of urgency as you have a suspected heart attack on your hands. When you get through, tell them that you are phoning on behalf of the patient, that they have had a suspected heart attack and that you have already phoned for the ambulance. Again, you may be asked a few questions, probably about the symptoms; answer them as clearly as you can. If you are phoning after surgery hours you may be put through to a duty doctor who doesn't know the patient, in which case you will be asked more questions, perhaps including where the address is and how to get to it; have a clear answer prepared if you can.

You may feel very nervous of taking control of the situation in this way, while at the same time very frightened about what is happening to the heart attack patient. Try and stay calm. The heart attack patient will also be frightened and may be in pain. If you panic you will not be able to help them.

Cardio-pulmonary resuscitation
If the patient has suffered a really serious heart attack they may have

stopped breathing and have no pulse. You can check this by carrying out the following.

- Lie the patient on their back.
- Turn the head to one side and clear any obstruction, e.g. vomit, from the mouth. Don't be squeamish, use your fingers and make certain there's nothing at the back of the mouth.
- Lift the chin and tilt the head back slightly.
- You can tell if they are breathing by placing your ear next to their mouth and listening carefully; watch their chest at the same time to see if it is rising and falling.
- Check their pulse at the wrist or the neck; for the neck pulse, move your fingers firmly round from the Adam's apple, under the chin, towards the bottom of the ear. The neck pulse should be about halfway round.
- If the pulse is faint or irregular, do not carry out the chest compression detailed below.

If there is no breathing and no pulse, one person should go immediately and phone for the ambulance and doctor, while another person carries out cardio-pulmonary resuscitation, as detailed below. If you are the only person with the patient and you can call out to others for help, carry out the cardio-pulmonary resuscitation, calling for help when you can; when others come, send them off to make the phone calls. However, if you are completely on your own and there is no one else around, go and contact the emergency services first. This is how to carry out the cardio-pulmonary resuscitation:

- Pinch the patient's nose shut, take a deep breath, put your mouth over theirs, ensuring that you make a good seal, and breathe slowly into their mouth. Their chest should rise.
- Lift your head away from their mouth, turning your head towards their chest, and breath in while watching their chest fall.
- Give them another breath into their mouth.
- Now give them 15 chest compressions. Find a point two finger-widths up from the base of their breastbone. Clasp your hands, fingers interlocked, palms away from you, arms straight. Place the palms on the point two finger-widths up from the base of the breastbone and press down firmly and quickly at a rate of slightly more than one a second (80 per minute).

- Give them two more breaths, then 15 more chest compressions.
- Continue with the 2:15 routine until the doctor or the ambulance arrive.

Cardio-pulmonary resuscitation is something that everyone can do. If you have someone in the family who is at risk of a heart attack, the whole family should learn how to do it. St John's Ambulance and other agencies can easily teach you – enquire at your health centre.

Once the emergency services get there

Once the paramedic or doctor has arrived they will assess the position. If a doctor is present and they think that a heart attack has occurred they will give the heart attack patient an injection of diamorphine (heroin). This is an opium-based drug, therefore:

- It gives rapid and effective pain relief. This will make the patient much more comfortable.
- It relaxes the patient and reduces their anxiety and fear about what is happening. This in turn reduces the risk of subsequent heart arrhythmias, when the electrical stimulation of the heart goes out of control.

When the ambulance arrives the patient will be carefully but swiftly put on a stretcher and carried into it. An oxygen mask will put on the face to help with breathing, and as soon as possible the ambulance will leave for the accident and emergency department of the nearest district general hospital. This will be an emergency journey and the blue lights will be flashing and the siren going.

As has already been explained, the heart attack patient is at risk of heart arrhythmias – the electrical stimulation of the heart goes out of control and the heart ceases to beat effectively, or it beats frantically fast and equally ineffectively. The first is known as *ventricular fibrillation* and the second tachycardia, and both tend to render the patient unconscious. If either of these happens it can be treated by a machine called a defibrillator. This has two handles that are pressed on to either side of the unconscious patient's chest; they deliver a charge of electricity across the chest and this can kick the heart back to beating properly. If it is necessary the ambulance crew may carry out this procedure as an emergency before putting the patient in the ambulance. If ventricular fibrillation occurs during the journey to the hospital they will be able to use the defibrillator in the ambulance.

You may be allowed to accompany the heart attack patient to hospital in the ambulance, but it is more likely that you will have to make your own way there. The ambulance crew have to be prepared for having to use the defibrillator; furthermore, there are many other uncomfortable heart arrhythmias, apart from ventricular fibrillation, which need urgent treatment with drugs. If the patient is not unconscious and needs treatment with the defibrillator, a light anaesthetic will have to be administered. Extra people in the ambulance could get in the ambulance staff's way, which is why you may not be able to travel with them.

In hospital

Arrival at hospital

Once the ambulance arrives at the accident and emergency department of the hospital the heart attack patient will be wheeled out of the ambulance and into the hospital as fast as possible. Events should then take place pretty swiftly, although as an onlooker they might sometimes seem to be agonisingly slow as discussions take place, tests are carried out and drips run up. In some cases the heart attack patient will be admitted directly to the cardiac/coronary care unit (CCU), in which case the treatment will be more efficient and swifter.

If the heart attack patient has not already received diamorphine, this will now be administered, along with aspirin to help reduce the risk of a further heart attack and to help dissolve the clot that has already blocked one or more of the coronary arteries. An ECG will be taken to determine exactly what has happened, and in some cases to make sure that a heart attack has occurred. A plastic cannula (a fine plastic tube) will be inserted into a vein in the patient's arm, and streptokinase will be administered via a drip into the arm. Streptokinase, as already mentioned, is a clot-busting drug that dissolves the clots that block the coronary arteries and cause heart attacks; it will reduce substantially the risk of a further heart attack. Indeed, the time from the first symptoms of a heart attack to the administration of streptokinase is now seen to be crucial; the shorter this time, the greater the chances of survival and of minimising the damage to the heart muscle. Hospitals are now working to reduce the door-to-needle time, i.e. the time it takes from entry into the accident and emergency department to the administration of streptokinase, by streamlining the admission of heart attack patients and getting their tests and assessments performed as swiftly as possible. Indeed, in very rural areas in particular there is now a strong argument for GPs to be in a position to administer streptokinase or other clot-busting drugs before the heart attack patient even enters the ambulance. You can do your bit by alerting the medical services as soon as you think a heart attack has taken place.

There are situations in which streptokinase cannot be administered:

- If the heart attack patient has suffered a recent stroke, had major surgery or is bleeding into the gut.
- If there is an active stomach ulcer.
- If the patient is pregnant.

If any of these circumstances apply there is a risk that the streptokinase will cause more problems than it solves and alternative clot-dissolving treatments will be used where possible. If streptokinase has been administered during the previous two years, alteplase, another clot-buster will be used.

If the heart attack patient is admitted to the accident and emergency unit, the streptokinase drip will be run up and the patient stabilised, perhaps with the administration of other drugs. They should then be transferred to the cardiac/coronary care unit – the CCU. If they are admitted directly to the CCU then the initial treatment will be decided more quickly.

But wherever the heart attack patient is admitted to, this early period is very harrowing, both for the patient and for whoever is accompanying them. There is the uncertainty surrounding the true nature of the symptoms, the phoning of the doctor and the ambulance – and if you are away from home or work this can pose a problem in itself – the rush to hospital and then the alien bustle and activity of the accident and emergency department. If you are accompanying the patient, try to stay with them as much as possible – it will provide a strand of contact with their normal life that is very valuable. There will be periods when you may not be able to stay right next to them, particularly if a crisis develops, but do try to make certain that the hospital staff are aware of your presence and of your desire to be with the patient.

The CCU
The coronary/cardiac care unit is basically an intensive care unit dedicated to cardiac patients, i.e. patients who have heart disease. There

may therefore be patients in the CCU who have had other heart problems, as well as heart attack patients. In most hospitals heart surgery patients are looked after on a separate cardiothoracic ITU and then a surgical cardiac ward. For most heart attack patients, the stay in the CCU will be for about two days – if no complications have arisen during this period it is unlikely that serious problems will arise during the rest of the stay in hospital, and they can therefore be safely transferred to the ordinary cardiology ward or a general medical ward. If there are complications, the heart attack patient will remain on the CCU for longer.

The CCU is a busy hi-tech environment, with all sorts of monitors and equipment hooked up to or plumbed into the patients. There is a lot of quiet bustle, with an incessant background bleeping of electronic monitors. To those who have never seen a CCU or an intensive care ward before, it can look more like something from a sci-fi movie.

To begin with you may be terrified by it, daunted by it, horrified by it or at best nervous within it. Gradually you get used to it, you begin to recognise faces, both of staff and other patients, and after a couple of days it all seems rather routine. Indeed, it might become quite exciting as you come to understand what is going on. There is always a fair bit of activity on a CCU, even during the night, with staff coming and going, monitors bleeping, the occasional monitor alarm going off, patients being checked regularly and every now and then a crisis with a patient. Night-time seems pretty much like daytime and you will probably find that your sleep pattern goes out of the window – you sleep a lot during the day, then lie awake bored out of your head during the night.

If you are a man you may well not have a pyjama top on; this is so that you don't have to take it off every time an ECG is taken, or when you have an examination. However, as the ward is kept at a constant warm temperature, this will not be a problem. You will be attached to a heart monitor, via pads and wires attached to your chest, and you will have regular ECGs taken to assess the state of your heart. For at least the early part of your stay on the CCU you will have a clear plastic oxygen mask on; the oxygen helps with breathing and pain reduction – as the blood takes in more oxygen than usual, so the heart doesn't have to make such an effort to get oxygen to the rest of the body. You will have a drip into your arm – a plastic tube leading into a plastic cannula that goes in a vein in your arm. To begin with, the clot-busting drug will have been run in through this drip, hooked up on to a drip stand by your bed. Later other drugs may be administered through it, but the drip will not be left up routinely. You may have a catheter going into your bladder – a small plastic tube allowing you to pee without noticing, the urine draining into a plastic bag under the bed.

You will not be left in bed for very long. As soon as the ward staff think it's suitable, probably within the first 24 hours on the unit, you will be helped out of bed. This might be for a bedside wash or to allow the bed to be made and you may find it tiring at first. To begin with you will find everything quite tiring, but the longer you are allowed to lie in bed the more out-of-condition your body becomes, the harder work you will find your rehabilitation and the slower will be your recovery. Some patients will not be allowed out of bed quite so quickly, for various clinical reasons – they may have other problems as well as having suffered a heart attack. Once they are ready, they will be got out of bed and their recovery will then proceed at the same pace as other patients.

Remember this word 'recovery'. You have had a heart attack, a section of your heart muscle has been damaged and will be scarred, and there may have been complications, but you are likely to recover. You will be walking around the ward within a few days, up and down a flight of stairs before you leave hospital, and if you are diligent about following an exercise programme after you leave hospital, you should be back at your normal level of fitness and activity, or better, within a few weeks. Getting out of bed is the first step on this road.

During your stay on the CCU you should be visited by a rehabilitation nurse and/or a physiotherapist. They will explain the hospital's heart attack rehabilitation programme and will encourage you to get moving as soon as you can – this not only means getting out of bed and getting walking as soon as possible, but also foot and arm movements while you are in bed, to assist the circulation and to keep your muscles and joints active. You should be taught some deep breathing exercises and encouraged to do these while you are lying in bed; these will exercise the chest and tummy muscles, and help to discourage any chest infections.

Nowadays, when you go into hospital, the hospital has a duty under the patient's charter to assign a named nurse to your care. This is as true of the CCU as it is of an ordinary ward. That nurse will be responsible for managing your care on that ward, and although they will not be on duty all the time, when they are on duty you will be under their care. Their name might be written on the wall above your bed and it will certainly be on a chart in the central administration area of the unit. This gives both the heart attack patient and their family and friends a point of contact, someone they can get to know and who can answer their questions or refer them on to other staff who are in a better position to answer questions. The nurse should introduce themselves to the patient as soon as the patient is in a fit state to register the information, and should certainly introduce themselves at the first opportunity to close friends and relatives of the patient. If you phone in to the ward wanting information, say who you are and who you are phoning about and ask if you can speak to the named nurse. If they are not on duty, ask to speak to whoever has taken over from them. If they are not available, ask to speak to the ward sister or the nurse in charge.

Visiting will probably be on an open basis, although there may be a limit on the number of visitors allowed at a bedside at any one time. If you want to stay by the bedside all day, holding the patient's hand perhaps, or gently talking to them as they drift in and out of sleep, that will probably be no problem. If it is, ask what the problem is. If you have specific questions about treatment, what's happening, the future, anything, start by asking the named nurse. They may well refer you on to one of the doctors. Trying to see hospital doctors, particularly registrars and consultants (the more senior doctors, whose name should be written on the wall above your bed), is not easy; although they will visit the CCU at least once on most days, they are busy, they have a lot of patients to look after, and on cardiac wards they are frequently dealing with emergencies. That having been said, though, they have a duty to explain to patients and close relatives what is going on and to answer questions. If you have difficulty getting to see the registrar or consultant, find out what their secretary's telephone number is (the nurse can find this out for you) and phone them during the day to make an appointment to see the doctor.

After a couple of days on the CCU, assuming there have been no problems, you will be moved to an ordinary cardiac ward or a general medical ward. This may well be quite worrying; 'What happens if something goes wrong?' 'Shouldn't I be monitored closely the whole time I'm in hospital?' 'I've got to know the people on the CCU – I don't want to move to another ward where I don't know anyone.' These, and other, fears and concerns are entirely to be expected, and everyone who has moved from a CCU to an ordinary ward has been through the same experience. Very simply, if you are being moved from the CCU to an ordinary ward it means that the crisis period after your heart attack has been safely passed and you are well on your way to recovery.

The cardiology/general ward

From the CCU your bed, drip and all if you've still got one, will probably be wheeled into the cardiology ward or the general medical ward, and your named nurse from the CCU will introduce you to and hand you over to your named nurse on the ward. This will be where you will stay for the rest of your time in hospital and, as with the CCU, you will quickly get used to who is who and what's where.

The first thing you will notice on the general ward is that there is less concentrated activity than on the CCU – it's not exactly a more relaxed place, but it's not such an intense atmosphere. It will get quite busy in the mornings as doctors do their ward rounds, checking up on the progress of their patients, beds are made, floors are cleaned, physiotherapists make their visits to patients and patients get up for washes, baths or showers. In the afternoons it will be quieter and you will undoubtedly want to rest. Nights should be more peaceful than on the CCU, and you should be able to get back to a pattern of being largely awake during the day and largely asleep during the night.

While you were on the CCU you will have been helped out of bed and into a chair on a number of occasions. You might have been helped to walk a few steps around the bed, trailing tubes and wires like an untidy heap of spaghetti. Now you are on the ward you will be expected to sit out of bed for increasing lengths of time – perhaps a couple of hours. You will be helped to walk to the end of the ward, perhaps to go to the loo. By day four or five in hospital you should be walking freely around the ward and the toilets, and you will probably have had a supervised bath or shower. And after that you can do as much walking as you feel capable of; certainly before you leave hospital you will have been taken up and down a flight of stairs by a nurse or physiotherapist to ensure that you can cope with stairs at home.

At the same time you will be disconnected from the bits of equipment and tubes. First to go will be the oxygen mask, then probably the urinary catheter if you had one. The heart monitor will obviously be taken off before you leave the CCU, and some time while you are on the cardiology ward the drip and needle in your arm will be removed. During your last day or so on the ward you may even be encouraged to get dressed during the day.

All this activity sounds fine and easy when described like this. In reality it will be absolutely exhausting. You will feel as weak as a kitten and will wonder if you will ever get your strength back. Everyone who goes through a heart attack feels equally exhausted. It does get better, your strength does return. If you are on day two or three in hospital and have just been pole-axed by a shuffle up and down the ward, look at the people who are waiting to go home, dressed and walking around the ward. They have only been in hospital a few days longer than you. In a week's time you will be in their position. Don't be downhearted. Make the effort to get on your feet and walk about, then use the time to rest and recover from it and recharge your energy reserves.

The CCU/cardiac ward will in many cases work with the rehabilitation staff as part of a team, but whatever the circumstance, during the time on the cardiology ward the rehabilitation nurse should come to see you and explain in more detail the rehabilitation and recovery programme that is available in the hospital. You will already have started on this rehabilitation programme on the ward, doing the movement and breathing exercises in bed and then walking progressively longer distances around the ward and perhaps up and down a corridor. You may well have received booklets and information sheets on what has happened to you, what is happening to you in hospital, what medicines you are taking and will be taking in the future, and about the rehabilitation programme that the hospital offers. This process of giving you information is part of the recovery programme; it helps you to understand what has happened to you, what has been done to you to help you recover, what is available in the future to help you and what you can do to help yourself. It will probably seem overwhelming at some stages – a mass of information to digest at the same time as you are trying to come to terms with a serious event in your life. Keep the information sheets and read them when you can concentrate on them, and ask questions if you don't understand anything. The ward nurses, and particularly the rehabilitation nurse, are there to help you recover and should make the time to answer your questions.

Many hospitals now run a 6- to 12-week rehabilitation programme for heart attack patients once they have left hospital and it is while you are still in hospital that this should be discussed with you. You must make every endeavour to get on such a programme; it will make an enormous difference to your recovery. If the places are limited, ask to go on a waiting list. If transport to and from the sessions is likely to be a problem, ask if any help is available. If no such recovery programme is available at the hospital, ask if one is available outside the hospital –

there may be GP organised schemes in some areas or your local leisure centre might run a properly supervised heart attack recovery programme.

Before you leave hospital you may be given an exercise ECG test, as already mentioned. To recap, this is like an ordinary ECG, but it is carried out while you are exercising. This means that the heart is monitored while it is carrying out some real work. It provides a lot more information about the health of the heart than an ordinary resting ECG. The exercise is provided by putting you on a treadmill – a short moving walkway that can be tipped up so that it seems as though you are climbing a hill – or on an exercise bike. You are connected up to an ECG and then told to walk or pedal for 5 to 10 minutes. To begin with it will seem relatively easy, but the load on the bike, or the slope of the treadmill, will gradually be increased until you are having to work quite hard. At the end of the test you will be sweating and breathless, but able to talk. It will be the most exhausting exercise you will have taken since your heart attack (and perhaps for a long time before), but the cardiac technician and doctor will ensure that it is well within your capability. Indeed, it should be a good indicator to you of what you can do without killing yourself; it is very common at this stage to fear that any exertion will bring on another heart attack. This test will show you that this is not the case. If possible, ask if your spouse or partner or a close family member can attend; they may be even more worried about what you can and can't do than you are, and it could be a very reassuring experience for them as well.

From the doctors' point of view, an exercise ECG will give a good idea of how much or how little the heart has been damaged by the heart attack. Any heart attack causes a certain amount of damage to the heart muscle – after all, the reason you had a heart attack was that a section of the heart muscle was starved of oxygen and nutrients by a clot blocking one of the coronary arteries. This damage to the heart muscle results in an area of scar tissue in the heart and, depending on its size, it will affect the functioning of the heart to a greater or lesser extent. The exercise ECG will also give the rehabilitation nurse a good idea of what level of exercise to start you on when you begin the rehabilitation programme.

Going home

After you have been in hospital for about a week you will be sent home. You have had a heart attack, you have got yourself back on your feet again, albeit helped by the health service. They can now do no more for you on an inpatient basis, and you are well enough to go home.

You will have got used to being looked after in hospital, you will still be taking on board the fact that you have suffered a life-threatening event, you will feel very wobbly and you will probably feel very, very nervous about going home. This is entirely understandable and is what most heart attack patients go through when they are discharged from hospital. However, if you are being sent home, then it means that:

- The hospital staff are perfectly confident that you can cope at home; they have ensured that you can walk around, that you can wash and bath yourself, that you can dress yourself, and that you can go up and down stairs.
- They will have asked about your domestic arrangements, and should have discussed them with you and your spouse or partner or a close family member.
- If there are domestic problems then the social services will have been involved if necessary and perhaps the health visitor contacted.
- You will have been given enough medicines to take home and to see you through the first week. It should have been explained to you what these medicines do, when you should take them and what to do if you forget to take one or take too many.
- You should have a note to take to your GP.
- You will probably have an outpatients appointment to come in to the clinic after a month or two.
- You should have a date to come into the rehabilitation classes in the hospital after about six weeks.
- You should have a sick note so that you can claim statutory sick pay or incapacity benefit.
- Arrangements should have been made for hospital transport if your family or friends can't take you home. You won't be allowed to drive yourself home, neither will the staff be keen for you to wander out of the hospital and catch a bus home.

If you have not received any of these by your final day in hospital or you are unhappy about any aspect of going home, discuss it with your nurse. Obviously you are not going to be able to stay in hospital an extra day or so just because you are nervous of going home, but the staff will make every effort they can to help you solve any problems that going home might raise and to make the transition from hospital to home as smooth as possible.

Surgery and other treatments and tests

As a result of your heart attack it might be necessary for you to undergo surgery or other follow-up tests and treatments. The details of what is involved with these – angiogram, angioplasty, stents and coronary artery bypass surgery – are covered in the previous chapter.

Urgent investigations and surgery

It is possible that while you are in hospital, if there is a cardiothoracic unit, you will have an angiogram carried out to assess the state of your heart function and to see how furred up your coronary arteries are. If this is necessary and possible, it is much more likely that it will be carried out while you are on the cardiology or general medical ward than on the CCU. Similarly, if it is decided that you need angioplasty or stents to stretch the blockages in the coronary arteries, and they can be carried out in the same hospital, these will probably be carried out while you are on the cardiology ward. It may mean that your discharge from hospital is delayed by a day or two, but it won't interfere with your recovery programme – it won't stop you walking around the ward or washing yourself, although it might mean a morning or a day without food and the sedation they give you for the investigations will leave you a little woozy for the rest of the day.

If it is decided that you need a coronary artery bypass operation as a matter of some urgency, then this will make a big difference to the length of time you spend in hospital. If the surgery is carried out while you are on the CCU, then you will spend quite a few days longer on the CCU or the cardiac surgery ward before being transferred to the cardiology or general medical ward. If you go for surgery once you have progressed to the cardiology ward, then you will end up back on the CCU or the cardiac surgery ward for a few days after surgery.

Once you come round from the anaesthetic after the operation you will find yourself linked up to all the tubes and machines already described earlier in the chapter. You will also have a tube in your mouth to help you with your breathing; remember that during the operation you will have been on a heart/lung bypass machine and after you come off it, while you are still under the anaesthetic, this assistance with your breathing is important. The tube will feel uncomfortable and will prevent you speaking properly, but it will be removed as soon as the nursing staff are happy that you can breathe successfully on your own.

You will have a line of stitches down your chest where the breastbone was opened up to give the surgeons access to your heart and, if the bypass blood vessels were taken from your leg, you will have stitches in your leg as well. You will be on fairly powerful pain relief, so although you will be aware of having undergone surgery and will not feel terribly comfortable, you will not be suffering from distressing pain. In fact at no stage should you be exposed to distressing pain; if you are, then the pain relief given to you is not doing its job and you should let the nursing staff know about it. There is absolutely no point in suffering pain; it tenses you up, dominates your thoughts and interferes with the healing process. Make use of the pain relief that is available and if it isn't working, whether it is during the day or night, tell someone. Suffering pain in silence is not a sign of strength, more a sign of stupidity, because you certainly aren't doing yourself any good.

After such surgery your time spent on the CCU or the cardiac surgery ward will be a day or so longer than if you'd merely had a heart attack. The physiotherapists will pay a bit more attention to you; during an operation there is a tendency for sputum to accumulate in the lungs and breathing tubes, and the physiotherapist will be keen to get you to do some deep breathing to help shift these accumulations and to get the lungs working properly. They will also show you how to cough without hurting the chest stitches.

You will be helped out of bed within two days of the operation, and possibly within a day of the operation, and after that your mobilisation will be as fast as anyone else who has just had a heart attack. When the CCU or cardiac surgery staff are satisfied with your progress and healing, you will be moved to the cardiology or general medical ward, and then your daily routine will be pretty much the same as everyone else. Perhaps the only difference is that you will be encouraged to keep your feet up when you are sitting or lying down, either on a stool or on a pillow on the bed. This is to prevent fluid collecting in the legs and causing swelling. You will also have elastic stockings to wear at all times, for the same reason – they do not look very elegant, but they make a big difference.

Towards the end of your stay in hospital the stitches will be removed from your chest and from your leg. The wound in the leg may weep for a day or so afterwards, especially if it is not kept raised when sitting or lying down, but if this happens a dressing will be applied to deal with it.

Rehabilitation after coronary artery bypass surgery is along the same lines as after a heart attack, although it may proceed more slowly. The rehabilitation nurse or physiotherapist will advise you on what to do when you get home and will book you onto any rehabilitation programme that the hospital runs.

Your discharge from hospital will be along exactly the same lines as for an ordinary heart attack patient.

Non-urgent investigations and surgery

Rather than an urgent investigation or surgery during your period in hospital immediately after a heart attack, it is more likely that you will be called back for tests on an outpatient basis and angioplasty, stents or coronary artery bypass surgery will be offered to you, if necessary, at a later date.

6 The longer term

When you arrive home from hospital you will probably be tired from the journey – just walking the short distance to and from the car will have made you feel very weary. You will also be very nervous. This is entirely normal and entirely understandable. You have suffered a life-threatening event, which, to say the least, is unsettling – it underlines your mortality and forces you to face facts that you may have ignored up until now. You have spent some time in hospital, which may have been another novel and rather unsettling experience. While you were in hospital your every need was looked after by someone else. Now, all of a sudden, you are back on your own again, with no nurse to call for if something goes wrong. For a time you will not be able to go to work, so the usual pattern of the day will have been lost. It can all be very worrying, even frightening.

What you must remember is that there are plenty of people to help you on your road to recovery. Accept the help that is offered, whether it is from the health service or from family, friends and neighbours. Find out what you can do to help yourself – ask questions, try and understand what has happened to you, and what you can expect to do at various stages of your recovery. Thousands of people a year have heart attacks and recover to lead perfectly healthy lives. You are no different from them.

What to expect of your GP

When you leave hospital you are handed over to the care of your GP. You will be going back to the hospital on an outpatient basis, for check-ups, tests and perhaps other procedures such as angioplasty, but your day-to-day care is now in the hands of your GP. You may not know them terribly well, although if you have a history of coronary heart disease there is a fair chance that you will have seen quite a lot of them, particularly if you have suffered from angina before having a heart attack. Over the next few months, though, you are going to get to know them quite well.

If you have an aversion to doctors, or are worried about bothering them, 'because they're always so busy', then you are going to have to learn to strike a balance. Your GP isn't necessarily going to be the key to your recovery, but they are in a position to help enormously. This does not just apply to the heart attack patient; a good GP will understand that the whole family has had a shock and that everyone is involved in the recovery process.

The first meeting with the GP

When you are discharged from hospital you will have been given a note for your GP. They will have been aware that you have had a heart attack, and may well have been in touch with the hospital to find out about your diagnosis and progress; ideally they should have been contacted by, or in contact with, the rehabilitation team at the hospital. However the GP will not know when you have been sent home until the note from the hospital is dropped off at your health centre or surgery, so someone needs to do this for you as soon as possible after you get home.

In an ideal world you should then receive a home visit from the GP within a week of being out of hospital. This has a number of advantages over a visit to see them at the health centre.

- The GP can allocate more time to see you, without the pressure of a waiting room full of other patients needing to be seen.
- They can talk to you in a relaxed atmosphere, in an environment where you feel comfortable.
- They can discuss details both with you and your spouse or partner or family.
- They can see what your home is like and identify any areas that might cause you problems during the first few days while you are still feeling weak and nervous.

When the note to the GP is dropped off at the health centre or surgery, whoever drops it off should ask the receptionist what the GP's policy is regarding visiting heart attack patients who have just been discharged from hospital. If they normally carry out a home visit in the first week out of hospital, all well and good. If they normally see heart attack patients in the first week but expect them to come to the health centre, ask if a home visit is possible, for all the reasons listed above. If an appointment is usual in the first week, but the receptionist is adamant that a home visit is not possible, make a health centre appointment, but ask for a longer one than usual because you have a lot of questions to ask. If an appointment in the first week is not usual, say that you would like one and that it would be useful if it were longer than usual because you have a lot of questions. At any appointment, whether it is at home or the health centre, emphasise that the spouse or partner or a close family member will be there – this is very important as the heart attack recovery process involves the whole family, not just the heart attack patient.

Before you see the doctor, write down a list of questions that you want to ask, whether they are about what happened to you during your heart attack, what happened to you in hospital, what's happening to you now or what you can expect in the future. By this stage in your recovery you will probably be brimming over with questions; don't feel nervous about asking the GP for the answers. And if you don't understand anything, ask again until you are clear about the answer.

The GP will have been told in the letter from the hospital precisely what drugs you are on. Tell them if you are suffering from any side-effects – odd feelings or a rash or a funny taste or bad dreams or difficulty sleeping can all be side-effects of some of the drugs you might be on, so mention them. It may be that a change from one drug to another will remove the side-effects.

Sooner or later you will need a repeat prescription for your medicines – the hospital will probably only have given you a week or two's worth. Sort out with the GP when you need to get some more and how they deal with repeat prescriptions at the health centre.

You will also need another sick note at some time. Discuss with the GP how long the hospital has signed you off sick and what you need to do when the sick note runs out.

Subsequent visits to the GP

Your GP will probably want to see you on a regular basis, perhaps once a month to begin with, to make sure you are recovering successfully and to deal with any problems that arise. It may be that when you need a repeat prescription or another sick note, this will be used as a reason for seeing you. These appointments will probably be at the health centre, unless there are serious reasons for the GP seeing you at home. After a month at home there should be no reason why you can't go to the health centre, even if you have to arrange transport there and back.

As with the first meeting with the GP, use subsequent appointments to ask questions and to clarify details. It cannot be emphasised enough that if you know what has happened, what is happening and what you can expect to happen, it puts you in a far more confident position to recover quickly and successfully from your heart attack and other symptoms of coronary heart disease.

Other services available through your health centre

Nowadays health centres are geared up to provide many services, and you should be prepared to make use of whatever you think might help you. There is a whole team working out of a typical health centre – often called the *primary healthcare team* – and you should come into contact with all of them during various stages of your recovery. Get to know them and learn about what they can offer.

- Most health centres now have at least one *practice nurse*. This does not mean they are practising to be a nurse. Far from it; they are fully qualified nurses, usually with other specific skills that allow them to assist the GPs and take on various functions that the GPs delegate to them. You will see quite a lot of the practice nurse – they will take blood samples from you, they may give you advice on diet, exercise and other aspects of your life, and they will be able to discuss with you the wider ramifications of your heart attack and how it is affecting you and your family.
- The *health visitor* might come in to see you at home. This will be to see how you are coping, whether you have any special needs, and generally to answer questions and make sure there are no problems. If such a visit does materialise (and you can't expect one in every part of the country) make certain that your spouse or partner or a close family member or friend is there as well, so that everyone's needs can be taken into account and dealt with.
- You might have been told by the hospital that you need to lose weight if you are to reduce your risk of another heart attack. If there is a *weight loss clinic* at the health centre, sign up for it. Don't worry if you are a man and the clinic seems to be full of women; they will probably welcome you with open arms. If you are unhappy about attending a clinic, talk it over with your GP or the practice nurse; they will be able to deal with the matter on an individual basis.
- If you are a smoker you will undoubtedly have been told by everyone to stop smoking. Easier said than done. See if there's a *smokers' clinic* at the health centre, and sign up for that as well. If there isn't, then the health centre staff can probably put you in touch with a

local group that can help. Again if you are unhappy about attending group sessions, discuss the matter with your GP or practice nurse.

- Some health centres organise a *group for people who have had heart attacks*. These can be very useful, especially in the early stages after a heart attack, as you can see how other people have recovered or coped with their difficulties. If the health centre doesn't have such a group itself, the staff may be able to put you in touch with outside support groups – many areas have such groups that come under the umbrella of the British Heart Foundation. If your health centre is no help, contact the BHF direct and ask about a local group.

- Some health centres have a *dietitian*. You will probably have received advice on what sort of foods you should be eating if you are to reduce your risks of another heart attack. If you are at all unclear about this, ask if you can see the dietitian, and make sure that you are accompanied by whoever does the cooking in the house.

- If you are having sexual problems, they might be due to side-effects of the drugs you are on. Discuss them with whoever you feel most comfortable with – your GP, practice nurse, health visitor or district nurse. If the problems are not to do with the medicines, there may be *counselling services* that you (and your partner) can be referred on to. It might be a relatively simple problem – weariness and fear of sex causing another heart attack – it might be more deep seated – marital problems that are exacerbated by the tension and worry of a heart attack. If you are to make a successful recovery from your heart attack, these problems will sooner or later have to be addressed and a good starting point is often at the health centre.

Don't be nervous about making use of all these services. They are all there for your benefit. If you attend the various groups and clinics, for a start you get out of the house (and discover that you *can* get out of the house without dropping dead). You also get to meet other people, some of whom have had the same problems as you and who have got over them or recovered from them, and who might be able to give you very useful advice and help.

GP-managed rehabilitation programmes

In some areas cardiac rehabilitation programmes are managed by the GPs rather than the district hospital. Usually they make use of the local leisure centre. This has the advantage that, as you then become fitter and stronger on the cardiac rehab programme, you are in a position to make use of the other facilities that the leisure centre has to offer – swimming, for example. If the rehab programme is GP-managed, you may already have been seen by someone from the programme while you were in hospital; they will have explained what the purpose of the rehab programme is, what it does, where it is run and when you can go along to it. If such a contact is not made in hospital, it will undoubtedly be raised when the GP first sees you.

Whatever else you do, you should make use of this programme and everything it offers. A well-managed cardiac rehabilitation programme, especially if it is in your area and easy to get to, offers you the best possible opportunity to recover successfully from heart attack. If getting to and from the rehab sessions is a problem, discuss this with the programme staff and see if arrangements can be made to help you. If no help is available with transport, check out public transport links or come to some arrangement with a friend or a relative to get you there and back.

What to expect of the hospital/specialist

When you leave the hospital to go home, it is like leaving somewhere safe and warm and supportive, somewhere where your every need is looked after, to be disgorged into the cold hostile outside world that all of a sudden seems strange and exhausting. In fact, although you've left the security of the ward, your links with the hospital and the staff you've got to know have not been broken completely.

Cardiac helpline
If you are lucky there will be a direct cardiac helpline. This will probably be run by one of the nursing staff and will be available if you have any panics – some symptoms that you're not sure about, what to do if you forget to take one of your medicines, for example. Before you leave the hospital you will be given the number and will probably have had a chat with the nurse who runs the helpline.

If you phone in with a problem or a query, you may get to speak to someone directly. If not, you will get an answerphone. Don't try to leave a long message. Tell them who you are, the time and date you are phoning and what your telephone number is, and ask them to phone back.

It has to be emphasised that, although this can be a very helpful facility, especially if you live on your own, it is not a service that many hospitals yet provide. If a named cardiac helpline is not available, then consider making use of the line to the cardiac/coronary care unit, the cardiology ward or the rehabilitation team.

Follow-up appointments

When you are discharged from hospital you will be given an appointment to attend the outpatient clinic in the hospital, probably four to six weeks later. After that the frequency of follow-up appointments will depend very much on the policy of the hospital and the speed at which you make a recovery. To begin with the appointments might be every month or two, but as time goes by they will decrease in frequency to every six months or even every 12 months.

To begin with at the outpatients clinic you may well be seen by the same doctors that you got to know on the ward, although as time goes by the junior doctors will change jobs and you will get to see new faces. This can be a little unsettling if you don't like change and can also be irritating if the new junior doctors insist on asking the same questions that the previous junior doctors asked. Be patient with them, they have a job to learn and they have to start somewhere. At other hospitals, though, it may well be that the outpatient clinic for you is run by another cardiologist-led team.

At the clinic you will be weighed and blood samples may be taken for various tests – a cholesterol test is a typical example. You will be asked various questions about your recovery, about any symptoms that are bothering you, how you are getting on with your medicines and whether they are causing any problems. You will have been advised in hospital about giving up smoking and what sort of foods to concentrate on if you are to reduce your risk of a subsequent heart attack. Your success on these fronts will be discussed with you, and further advice given if necessary.

The doctor will also discuss with you whether you need to come into hospital for follow-up tests such as an angiogram, which would help determine whether you need follow-up procedures such as angioplasty, the insertion of a stent or coronary artery bypass surgery. If such tests or procedures are necessary you will either be given an appointment while you are at the clinic or the hospital will contact you by post at a later date. The length of time you have to wait for such an appointment will reflect in part the length of waiting lists at that hospital and in part the degree of urgency attached to your case.

Exercise ECG

The exercise ECG test has been described in the previous chapter. You may have such a test while you are in hospital, before you are sent home. It is equally possible that you will undergo such a test about four to six weeks after the heart attack. If you are going on to a rehabilitation programme, you will undoubtedly have such a test, as the results form the basis on which your initial exercise programme will be based. Furthermore, such a test will be carried out if a decision has to be made on whether to offer you surgery or angioplasty.

At this stage in your recovery you might be walking around the house and garden quite happily, or making short journeys to the shops, but you might be nervous of doing anything more energetic in case you further damage the heart. The exercise ECG will show you that you can push yourself quite hard with no disaster. If possible, ask if your spouse or partner or a close family member can attend the test; they may be even more worried about what you can and can't do than you are, and it could be a very reassuring experience for them as well.

Rehabilitation programme

The majority of cardiac rehabilitation programmes are based in district general hospitals, usually in the physiotherapy gym. Some of them are very small, with perhaps only 10 people on the course at any one time, and some are massive. Most cater for 10–20 people at a time on a 6–12 week rolling programme. Unfortunately, in some hospitals there are no rehabilitation programmes at all, but this problem will be discussed later in the book in the chapter on exercise.

If there is a hospital rehabilitation programme you will probably have been visited by the programme coordinator (usually a cardiac nurse or sister, or a physiotherapist) while you were in hospital, and given a date when you can attend your first session. If not, you will probably have been informed of your first session by post or, at the latest, at your first follow-up outpatients appointment.

Unfortunately, some heart attack patients are felt to be not suitable for a place on a rehab programme. For example, some programmes weed out what they see as 'high risk' patients, while others will not let anyone over 70 onto their programmes. Usually this weeding out process reflects the fact that the programme has only a limited number of places on it and the staff want to keep them for those they think will benefit most. However, there is strong evidence that the majority of people who suffer heart attacks (or have had heart surgery) benefit from a cardiac rehab programme, so if you find you have been excluded from such a programme, ask why and whether an exception can be made in your case.

Just as with a GP-managed rehab programme, make every effort to get on to a hospital-based cardiac rehabilitation programme; it offers you the best possible opportunity to recover successfully from a heart attack. If getting to and from the sessions is a problem, discuss this with the programme staff and see if arrangements can be made to help you. If no help is available with, see what public transport links there are, or try to come to some arrangement with a friend or a relative to get you there and back.

What to expect of yourself

When you come home from hospital after a heart attack you will feel a very different person from the person you were before the heart attack. Although you might have been aware that you suffered from some of the symptoms of coronary heart disease, everyone always thinks that heart attacks are like car accidents – they happen to someone else.

You will feel weak and helpless, frightened that you might never be able to work again and undermined by having had a brush with death. You will have had enough time in hospital – perhaps your first stay in hospital ever – to have become institutionalised; you'll have got to know the staff and the other patients, you'll have got used to the routine, have been able to chat about treatments and recovery and other people's illnesses. Now all of a sudden you are back home and it's all very strange.

Caution
To begin with you will probably be very cautious, for fear that any exertion will trigger another heart attack. At its worst this may cause you to stay in bed late and to move from bed to armchair, in front of the TV, then back to bed at the end of the day.

It may also be a strange situation you have come home to. You will have been used to going off to work every day; being around the house all day, particularly during weekdays, will be very unsettling. If you are a man, your wife or partner will have her routine for the day and you will not be used to it. You may be nervous of interfering with this routine or may simply feel excluded. If you are a woman and a house-wife, it will be even worse because you will be at home but will have to accept some help with the housework, from people who don't know your routine. You may be eager to get back to the looking after the house, but, again, very nervous of overdoing it.

Anxiety

Anxiety is always a major problem on coming home. This is due to all sorts of questions and fears.

- First and foremost, there is the fear of another heart attack. For some people this can dominate their lives, particularly as, once they are at home, they know that they don't have the hospital staff at hand to step in if there is an emergency.
- Then there is the anxiety relating to work. 'Will I ever be able to work again?' 'Will I be able to do the housework?' 'Will I be able to do the same work?' This fear looms much larger in the minds of younger people and those who have active jobs.
- This feeds into anxiety about finances. If you are of working age, for a while after a heart attack you will be off work and on statutory sick pay or incapacity benefit, both of which may bring in less than you've been used to. If you are worried about being able to go back to work, or back to the same work, there will be the fear of a long-term reduction in income.
- You may be worried about whether you will be able to continue with your leisure activities. 'Who will do the garden?' 'Should I stop going to the pub?' 'Can I get back to playing golf/tennis/bowls/whatever?'
- You might be worried about how your friends and colleagues are going to view you now. 'Will they see me as half the man I used to be?'
- And, underlying all these anxieties and fears, there will your own view of yourself. 'Am I an invalid now?'

These and many more anxieties and questions and worries will settle on your shoulders when you get home. This is entirely understandable and happens to everyone who's had a heart attack. You are not on your own, and talking to others at rehabilitation sessions will reveal this, help to solve problems and make you a lot more comfortable psychologically.

Some of the anxieties are justifiable and will need addressing in the future. Some worries will be completely unnecessary and as time passes they will be revealed as such. The important point to remember is that, yes, you have had a heart attack and it is a serious event. But the risk of another heart attack diminishes rapidly after the first day after the first heart attack; the very fact that you have been sent home is an indication that the doctors know you are well on the road to recovery. If your heart has suffered serious damage as a result of the heart attack you may not be able to recover to the level of activity you were used to, but for the majority of heart attack patients there is no reason why you cannot recover to the same or better levels of activity.

You were ill, you are recovering and you will be well again – that is the basic truth you have to fix in your mind.

Depression

Homecoming depression affects the majority of heart attack patients and for most it can be very unsettling. You might be nervous about leaving hospital, but everyone – you, your family, your friends – will also be excited that you are able to come home. Then you sit down, and this wave of anxiety pours over you, and you burst into tears. And you don't burst into tears once – it seems to happen all the time. And you become irritable, snapping at people at the slightest provocation. You feel awful. Is this the result of the heart attack? Has your mind in some way been damaged by it?

The answer is no. Depression – for that's what it is – is a perfectly normal part of recovering from any kind of serious illness or life-threatening emergency. You would go through the same depression if you had been in hospital after a car accident. The depression will last a few days, maybe a week or so, then you will pull out of it perfectly easily as you recover your strength and resume your normal activities.

If you feel that the depression is getting worse or going on for too long, tell your GP or phone the cardiac helpline to the hospital if there is one or tell the district nurse, but tell someone. Abnormal depression occurs in very few heart attack patients; it can be treated very effectively, but only if you tell someone.

Denial

Some heart attack patients cope with the whole situation by denying that anything serious at all has happened. They get home, they immediately do all the chores they were used to doing, they roar off down the pub with their friends, they rush around mowing the lawn, and shout and snap at anyone who tries to persuade them that they are doing too much. It is almost as if they are testing fate.

This may lead to them going back to work as soon as possible and picking up the same pressured work patterns that may have led to the first heart attack. Some heart attack patients have even been known to start dealing with work while they were still in hospital, getting their secretary to come in with files, dictating letters, making phone calls.

Surprisingly, there is no clear evidence to show that such inappropriate behaviour increases the immediate risk of another heart attack. What is a problem is when such behaviour leads to a refusal to heed the advice on how to reduce the long-terms risks of subsequent heart attacks. 'No I'm not going to give up smoking, I'm not going to take exercise, I don't care if I'm overweight, I'm not going to change my diet. I'm perfectly all right, if only you'd stop pestering me.'

This sort of angry denial that there is anything wrong is a means of coping with the facts, but it is not a successful or satisfactory way, and may only be ended by another heart attack. If this sort of behaviour is apparent in the heart attack patient, it is invariably difficult to discuss it with them. The advice is for the spouse or partner or a close family member to raise the matter with the GP or someone from the cardiology ward or clinic and to ask what can be done to help.

Determination to recover

Perhaps the most important ingredient in the recipe for recovery after a heart attack is determination, tempered with the understanding that recovery is a progressive process that will give rise to permanent lifelong changes. You are not ill one day and well the next day: you are ill one day and will be well a few weeks later if you are prepared to do a bit more each day.

You will increase your chances of recovery if you understand what has happened to you and what you need to do to rectify the problems that led up to the heart attack. Read as much as you can about heart disease, heart attacks and aids to recovery – the more you know, the more you will understand about what the recovery process involves. You can then make your own decisions, which makes you feel more in control of the situation, which in turn increases your self-confidence and will to succeed.

When you were in hospital you spent a lot of time in bed while your body healed itself. It only takes a few days of bed-rest for your body to get out of condition; if you were relatively weak and unfit before your heart attack, you will be very weak and unfit when you come home. Any exercise, even walking around the house, will make you puff and blow, make you feel tired, make your heart race or even skip a beat. This is entirely normal; anyone who is as unfit and weak as you are will have the same physical response as you. The biggest mistake is to feel that non-stop rest and peace and quiet are somehow restorative; they are not. Indeed, non-stop rest will make your recovery even more slow and laborious. Feeling puffed if you help clear the table after a meal on your first day home is entirely to be expected. When you help clear the table the next day you will feel less puffed, so perhaps you can help with the washing up as well. Do a bit more around the house each day until you are back to your usual chores. You have to realise that if you are to recover you must be prepared to make an effort every day. Don't indulge in a burst of activity that leaves you so breathless that you can't talk – that would be overdoing it. But there is nothing wrong with feeling weary.

When you do feel weary, take a break. Listen to your body. You will need to sit and snooze every now and then. Spending the whole day in bed or in an armchair is going to do you no good at all, but having a nap after lunch or even in the middle of the morning will do you no harm. Don't feel guilty about it, either. Your body is busy healing itself and periods of rest and relaxation are necessary. As you recover your normal levels of activity the need for these naps and snoozes will reduce, but when you need them don't ignore the message.

After a heart attack you are surrounded by people who want to help you get better – the health service, your family, your friends, your neighbours. They will all do what they can and some will be more help than others. But the most important person in your recovery is you. First you must understand and accept that you will recover. Then you must understand that you will be the key individual in this process and that if you are determined to recover you are halfway there.

But you must beware of becoming like… let's call him Mr Smith, RIP. He had a heart attack, he survived it, he came out of hospital and did all the right things – he gave up smoking, took regular exercise, changed his eating habits, got his weight down. Everything went fine for a year or two, then gradually he began to slip back into his old ways: the occasional cigar, then cigarettes; less and less exercise; his weight started to go back up; his blood cholesterol level, which he'd managed to get down to a low level, started to climb again. Four years after his first heart attack he had his second and this one was fatal – he was dead by the time he arrived at hospital.

Sex

Sooner or later after a heart attack you will start wondering about sex. 'Can I have sex again?' 'When can I have sex again?' 'Will I have a another heart attack if I have sex again?' 'Will everything work as normal?'

In some cases a heart attack can improve a couple's sex life. It brings them closer together, this improves the overall relationship and a better sexual relationship is part of this improvement. However, it has to be said that such couples are in the minority.

The main problem areas are as follows – everyone who has had a heart attack faces these at some stage:

- Fear that sexual intercourse will bring on a heart attack.
- Fear that sexual activity is somehow more likely to bring on a heart attack than other activity.
- Inability to relax because of the fear of a heart attack.
- Loss of desire for sex.
- Too tired for sex – you go to bed and promptly go to sleep.
- Impotence or inability to ejaculate (to come) in men; loss of sexual desire in women and vaginal dryness.

This last reason may be due to anxiety or exhaustion, but is more likely to be a side-effect of the drugs you are on. If this is a problem, pluck up the courage to discuss it with your GP or at the cardiac clinic. It is a problem that is well recognised, and can usually be solved by changing your medicines.

As regards activity levels and attached risk, sexual activity is exactly the same as any other activity (although one would hope more pleasurable) – it raises the pulse rate, i.e. the number of times the heart beats per minute. During sex the heart rate goes up to about 120 beats per minute. This is roughly equivalent to climbing two flights of stairs. So, if you feel your heart can cope with two flights of stairs then it can cope with sexual intercourse.

If sex brings on angina pain, treat the pain as you would angina pain at any other time – take a nitrate tablet or spray. If you know that sex brings on angina pain, don't stop having sex, simply take a nitrate pill or spray before you have sex. If angina pain is a problem, though, tell your GP. You will probably be getting angina from other activities as well and the GP needs to know about this in case you need to go for an angiogram or further treatment.

Sex may well be a problem because you or your partner are nervous about what it will do to you. Take it slowly, try it when you have some energy for it and are not exhausted, and don't worry if it is not terribly satisfactory to begin with. It will get better as you get used to it again.

Many younger people think that older people don't have sex, or don't have much sex. Heart attacks tend to happen to older people. Doctors and nurses tend to be younger people. Therefore, if you have problems or worries about sex and you discuss it with a nurse or doctor or other health worker, you might not get what you feel to be a satisfactory response. Try not to be put off; if your GP doesn't appear to take the problem seriously, bring it up with the cardiac clinic staff, or vice versa, or have a talk with the district nurse if they are coming to see you. Some health centres can put you in touch with someone who deals with sexual problems – ask if there is such an individual. Relate (formerly the Marriage Guidance Council) can also help – their telephone number will be in the telephone directory.

What to expect of others

So far we have looked at what you can expect of yourself, the sort of problems you are likely to come up against and the manner in which you might react to them. But what about other people – your wife or husband, other members of your family, friends? How are they likely to react, what problems are they likely to pose and how can they best be dealt with?

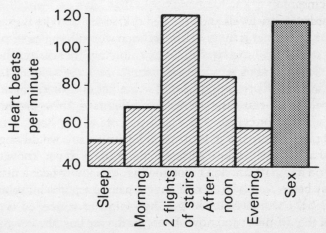

Fig. 9 *Heart rate in beats per minute for various activities, including sex.*

Spouses' and family needs

To begin with, it has to be accepted that, just as the heart attack patient has various needs – the need for information, the need for reassurance, the need for a clearly defined path to recovery – the spouse or partner of a heart attack patient and the close family also have needs. Often these are ignored or unmet, and this can have a very significant impact on the chances of a successful recovery from the heart attack.

- First and foremost, the spouse or partner will want to be considered, included and involved in the care and recovery of the heart attack patient. If you feel you are being excluded, by ward staff, by hospital doctors or by your GP, say so. Make certain you are present at as many appointments as possible that the patient has, whether they are in hospital, at the clinic, at home or at the health centre. If a cardiac rehabilitation programme is available, find out if you can go along to see what's happening and to talk to the staff about what you can do to help.
- Spouses and partners need information. They are not ill, and can read and digest information more rapidly and successfully in the early stages of recovery. Try and get copies of all the information sheets and booklets that the heart attack patient is given, and if you don't understand them, ask someone to explain them. Many district hospitals now have health information 'shops'; if you are lucky enough to have one at your hospital, go in there and ask what they've got on coronary heart disease and heart attacks. Go to your library or bookshop and ask what books they have on heart disease and heart attacks.
- A spouse or partner is invariably very keen, right from the start, to do as much as they can to reduce the risk of another heart attack. Again, this comes down to information and advice – make sure you are included in all consultations, that you get all the information sheets, that you see the cardiac rehab team and the dietitian.
- Spouses and partners need as much support as the heart attack patient. This can be from within the health and social services – particularly if you have a job that you are reluctant, or cannot afford, to give up. If you are in this position, go to your health centre as soon as possible and find out what is available, or ask the ward staff for help and advice. Often, though, what is needed is the opportunity to talk to a wife or husband who has already been through a similar experience of caring for a heart attack patient.

Again, ask at your local health centre or ask the ward staff if they can suggest someone. The British Heart Foundation keeps a register of clubs and groups of people who have had heart attacks – if there is a group near you, get in touch with them as soon as possible.

On discharge from hospital, it is important that the spouse and close family of the heart attack patient should understand the following:

- What has happened, i.e. do you understand what the heart attack did to the patient?
- What are the risk factors that gave rise to the heart attack, i.e. smoking, lack of exercise, high blood pressure, overweight, etc.
- What has been done and will be done by the hospital and health service to help the patient recover from the heart attack.
- What medicines have been prescribed, when they should be taken, how to get more of them, and what their side-effects might be.
- What exercise is recommended at different stages during recovery.
- When sexual activity can be resumed and what the problems might be.
- What the cardiac rehabilitation programme involves, where it is, when it is, when to begin attending, etc.
- Addresses and telephone numbers if advice or help is needed.

If you are fortunate enough to be reading this before discharge from hospital, make sure these points are clarified for you. If the heart attack patient is already at home and there are questions that still need answering, get on to someone – your GP, the cardiac clinic staff, the cardiac helpline if there is one, and try and get the answers.

Over-protection

Many wives and husbands of heart attack patients – particularly the wives – can become over-protective. This is partly driven by guilt; they somehow feel guilty that they have been in part responsible for the heart attack. 'Should I have "forced" my husband to work so hard?' 'Should I have expected so much of him around the house?' 'Have I nagged him too much?' 'Should I have been preparing healthier food?' 'Should I have made an effort to get him to give up smoking or drinking?' 'Should I have contacted the doctor sooner when he had a heart attack?' These and all sorts of other questions may be milling around in the partner's mind. This is all a perfectly normal reaction, and is very common. The answer to all the questions is probably 'No', but it doesn't stop the spouse or partner from feeling that they must somehow wrap the heart attack patient in cotton-wool and prevent them from undergoing anything strenuous or stressful. Any sort of physical exercise by the heart attack patient is discouraged, children and other family members are told not to make a noise or cause any fuss, anything that might lead to an argument is avoided – in short, life takes on a stressfully abnormal feeling. In some cases this involves the spouse or partner never leaving the heart attack patient unattended.

The whole family must understand that the heart attack patient has been treated in hospital for the heart attack and has been sent home because they are well on the road to recovery. To begin with their strength will be down, and they will still need rest to help them recover. However they need encouragement to get back to a normal life. They need to be encouraged to do a little more each day, to extend their levels of activity, gradually to resume a normal life.

Where the spouse or partner finds it very difficult to let the heart attack patient do anything that is seen as strenuous or stressful, despite assurances, discussion and advice, the problem can sometimes be unstuck by agreeing a 'contract'. The couple decide on activity – a walk down the road and back, say – and agree between the two of them what it is going to involve and how long it is going to last. For example, it might be a walk down the road that lasts no longer than 10 minutes. Both partners have to agree to this contract; the heart attack patient has to walk (no running) and has to be back in 10 minutes, while the spouse or partner has to stay in the house and not interfere (no phoning neighbours or craning out of the window). If this is successful, perhaps a 15-minute walk might be tried the next day, or two 10-minute walks, one in the morning and one in the afternoon. The two important features of this 'contract' are that both partners agree to the terms and the terms are strictly adhered to.

If this approach is adopted seriously and sensibly, then it can help deal with the problem of over-protection. If this does not seem like a good idea, or if it doesn't work, and over-protection seems to be getting in the way of recovery, a discussion with the GP or with staff at the cardiac clinic should take place. It must be understood that recovery is dependent on doing a little bit more each day, making a greater effort each day and exercising until you do feel weary. Far from killing you, this is going to save your life.

Denial

In contrast to the previous section on over-protection, some spouses and families indulge in a form of denial. This seems more likely to occur when the heart attack patient is a woman. The spouse or partner refuses to accept the fact that a heart attack is a serious event and assumes that, if the heart attack patient has been discharged from hospital, she is well enough to take on the all the work around the house that she's always done – cooking, washing up, cleaning, washing, the lot. Exhaustion sets in before the first day is even part way through, inducing anxiety and worry.

It must be remembered that all activities, from washing up to formal exercise programmes, should be taken up or resumed on a gradual and systematic basis.

Practical details

The following section offers some practical details that need considering or acting on when you go home from hospital after a heart attack.

Symptoms – what to expect

The following symptoms are entirely normal and need not be worried about:

- Tiredness.
- Light-headedness.
- Left-sided chest pain, either sudden or niggling.
- Skipped heart beats or extra heart beats.

The following symptoms may be more serious and you should let your GP or cardiac clinic know if you get any of them:

- Breathlessness after the smallest exertion.
- Breathlessness at night that wakes you up.
- Rapid thumping in the chest, especially if you feel faint at the same time.
- Chest pain, that may involve the neck and arms, that comes on with exercise or exertion and goes away with rest.
- Chest pain, that may involve the neck and arms, that comes on at rest and that is not helped by nitrate tablets or spray.

Using glyceryl trinitrate

Glyceryl trinitrate tablets and sprays – otherwise known as GTN, Isordil and Sorbitrate, isosorbide dinitrate, Ismo 20 or Monit, isosorbide mononitrate – are prescribed to control the symptoms of angina. To recap, the symptoms of angina are a tightness or band around the chest; a gripping pain in the chest; a feeling of oppression in the chest; pain in the arms, especially the left arm, that may run down to the wrist and hand; pain in the neck and chin. This pain comes on with exercise or exertion and goes away when you stop the exercise and rest; sometimes it can come on at rest.

If you have had a heart attack, you will probably be prescribed nitrate tablets or sprays. If they are to be effective, you must use them properly:

- When you get angina pain (as detailed above), place a nitrate tablet under your tongue or puff the spray under your tongue. This should relieve the pain within a few minutes.
- If the pain is not relieved within five minutes of taking the first tablet or spray, take a second tablet or spray.
- If the pain is not relieved within another five minutes, take a third tablet or spray.
- If the pain is not relieved within another five minutes, phone your GP immediately; it does not matter what time it is, phone the doctor.
- If you know that exercise or exertion is likely to bring on the angina pain, e.g. walking up a hill, take a nitrate tablet or spray beforehand. This is very important; many people do not realise that they can do this.
- There are a number of side-effects to nitrate tablets and sprays (see Chapter 4, page 49). If you get dizzy or a thumping headache after taking a tablet, spit out the tablet. Tell your doctor when you next see them.
- Nitrate tablets go off after six to eight weeks. Always keep them in the brown bottle they come in, with the top screwed on tight. If they are six weeks old, tell your doctor or the health centre, ask them for a repeat prescription and as soon as you get the new ones, throw the old ones away.
- Nitrate sprays do not go off until they are two years old.

Benefits

When you leave hospital you will have been given a sick note, sometimes called a medical certificate. This will probably be for a month.

- Make a note of when your sick note runs out. A day or so before this date you will need to ask your GP for another one. You might only need to let the receptionist at your health centre know you need another sick note; they may be able to get your GP to write one for you to collect from the health centre.
- If you work for an employer you may be entitled to statutory sick pay, in which case you need to send your sick note to the personnel office at your employer's.
- If you are unemployed or self-employed or you cannot get statutory sick pay you are entitled to claim Incapacity Benefit, in which case you need to fill in form SC1 from the Benefits Agency (part of what used to be the DHSS).
- If you are at all unsure about what you are entitled to, you or your family must contact the Benefits Agency either in person or by phone. They are listed in the business numbers section (the first section) of your phone book, under Benefits Agency, and there will undoubtedly be a full-page advertisement for them on a facing or following page. Do not be nervous about contacting them; they will be friendly and helpful.
- The Benefits Agency will be able to tell you about any other benefits you might be entitled to, such as income support, help with NHS charges, housing benefit and council tax benefit.

Work

For many people who have had a heart attack, one of their principal concerns is whether or when they will be able to return to work. For a few it is difficult to return to work; airline pilots and LGV (used to be called HGV) drivers usually find it impossible to return to their previous work, simply because they usually lose their licence. However, a few are allowed back to work after a satisfactory exercise ECG test. Others may think that it will be hard to return to work because their work involves a degree of manual labour; however, with a rehabilitation programme and a good progressive exercise regime, this should not necessarily be the case. This is something that you should discuss with the cardiac rehabilitation coordinator or your GP or at the cardiac clinic.

You might think that it will be risky to go back to work because it is a high-stress occupation. However it is perfectly possible to learn techniques to reduce or cope with stress; cardiac rehabilitation courses should be able to help you, as can stress management courses.

Whatever you do, do not write yourself off too quickly; a hasty decision to give up work might well be regretted later, when it's too late to do anything about it.

Many people do not go back to work after a heart attack, not because they are physically unfit for work, but because of fear or anxiety or some other deeper psychological reason. As this book has tried to emphasise all along, if your heart has not suffered serious damage as a result of the heart attack, it is reasonable to expect to achieve a level of fitness and activity that is at least as good as you had before the heart attack and in most cases that is better and healthier. This means that there is often no reason why you cannot return to your old job, provided you have the will and determination to do so. If this is what you want to do:

- Discuss it with your GP, the staff at the cardiac clinic and on the cardiac rehabilitation programme and see what help and advice they can give.
- If you work for an employer, visit the personnel office and discuss the matter with them.
- In some circumstances it might possible to move to a less arduous or less stressful job, either within your original workplace or organisation, or by moving to another workplace or organisation. It may involve a drop in salary or wages; if the opportunity looks attractive, sit down and see if you and your family will be able to live on the lower income.
- If you are self-employed, look carefully at what you do and what you might be able to do to make the work less stressful or less physically arduous.

However, it is also the case that many people who have had a heart attack use the event as an opportunity to take early retirement or redundancy. If you do not enjoy your work, particularly if you are close to retirement age, see if this is possible:

- Staff at the Benefits Agency will be able to advise you on what long-term benefits might be available to you if you choose this option.
- If your GP is prepared to sign you off long-term sick, it might make this option somewhat simpler. Discuss this with them.
- Go and talk to your personnel office or your manager at work. They

might be quite keen for you to take early retirement or some sort of redundancy package.

Perhaps the most important piece of advice is to sit down with your spouse or partner and close family and discuss the matter is some detail before coming to a firm a decision one way or another. When you are in hospital, or when you first come home, you might desperate to get back to work – you have lost your health, you don't want to lose your work, your identity, as well. Or perhaps, in contrast, you are desperate not to go back to work, but are nervous about what the financial implications might be or what people's reactions might be. All this needs to be discussed, however hard it might seem to bring the subject up.

Driving
If you have an ordinary driving licence then the following conditions apply, and must be understood.

- If you have had a heart attack or coronary artery bypass surgery, you shouldn't drive for a month after the events. You can retain your driving licence, though, and don't need to notify the Driving and Vehicle Licensing Agency (DVLA) in Swansea. (You ought to write to your insurance company, though, as they may well require more details.)
- If you have had angioplasty (and this will include having a stent fitted) you should not drive for a week after the procedure. Again, you can retain your licence and don't need to inform the DVLA.
- If you suffer from angina that occurs when driving you are advised not to drive and you must inform the DVLA.
- If you suffer from angina that only occurs on exercise you can retain your licence and need not inform the DVLA.

The DVLA's Driver's Medical Unit (see next to DVLA in the Useful Addresses at the end of the book) should be contacted for more detailed information.

If you hold a Large Goods Vehicle (LGV, formerly HGV) or a Passenger Carrying Vehicle (PCV, formerly PSV) licence and you have had a heart attack, suffer from angina, hypertension, arrhythmias or ECG abnormalities, or have had angioplasty (including the insertion of a stent) or coronary artery bypass surgery, then you should notify the DVLA. In the past, having a heart attack or a heart problem would automatically disqualify your licence. Nowadays the situation is not so harsh, but it is complex.

Depending on the problem, you may be disqualified from driving on the LGV or PCV licence for a period from a few weeks to a few months. But providing you can fulfil certain exercise or health criteria, you will get your licence back after the disqualification period has run out.

If you hold an LGV/PCV licence and you have had a heart attack, contact the DVLA's Drivers Medical Unit, explain your situation and ask for information sheet CLE1111. When you receive this sheet there will be medical sections that you probably won't understand; discuss the situation with your GP or at the cardiac clinic. They will be able to explain things simply to you and book you for the specific medical tests that you need to go through if you want to hold on to your licence.

7 Exercise

Various definitions of cardiac rehabilitation have been put forward. The World Health Organisation have suggested that it is:

> The sum of activities required to influence favourably the underlying cause of the disease, as well as to ensure the patients the best possible physical, mental and social conditions so that they may, by their own efforts, preserve, or resume when lost, as normal a place as possible in the life of the community.

This definition assumes an 'active and productive life' within the community, and this in turn is dependent on the adoption and maintenance of a lifelong pattern of exercise. This pattern of exercise:

- Begins when you are in hospital after a heart attack – *Phase 1*.
- Should be increased when you go home – *Phase 2*.
- Will be further developed by whatever rehabilitation programme is available to you – *Phase 3*.
- Should then continue for the rest of your life – *Phase 4*.

The whys and wherefores of exercise

This section will explain what exercise is and what it does for you. Later sections will explain specifically what should be available and what you can do at different stages of your recovery from a heart attack.

Why exercise?
This is perhaps the most important chapter in the book, for it is through regular exercise that you stand the best chance of resuming an active life and of preventing further heart attacks and reducing the symptoms of heart disease. To begin with it is useful to explain exactly why exercise is so important. If you understand the theoretical benefits of exercise, even if only simply, the reasons for taking up and continuing exercise will become more relevant to you.

- Exercise should improve your stamina – your ability to undertake an activity for a length of time without getting tired, e.g. walking for two hours. For this you must take regular aerobic exercise, i.e. exercise that leaves you puffed out and that uses large groups of muscles in a continuous, dynamic and rhythmic way. Walking, jogging, cycling and swimming are good examples of aerobic exercise.
- Exercise should improve your strength – your ability to undertake heavier activities, e.g. lifting a dustbin, carrying a shopping bag.
- Exercise should improve your flexibility – your ability to bend and turn and stretch, e.g. bending down to weed the garden.

But how are all these benefits gained? What does exercise do to your body that is so beneficial? To explain this we need to go back to basics. The body needs oxygen. The blood picks up oxygen in the lungs. The heart then pumps this blood around the body, and the body, e.g. the muscles, removes this oxygen from the blood and makes use of it. When you take more activity the body needs more oxygen and the heart has to pump faster to get the blood to the muscles. If you take very little exercise, every bit of exercise, e.g. climbing stairs, is going to make a heavy demand on your heart and if it is diseased it will complain (angina) or suffer damage (a heart attack). If you regularly take exercise and gradually increase the amount of exercise you take each day, the body responds to this work by working more efficiently.

What we are looking at in this chapter are exercises that are linked together into programmes that will get your body and heart back to, or in most cases better than, the levels of activity and stamina that you were accustomed to before your heart attack. There are three principles underlying such programmes.

- **Overload** To gain improvement muscles must be asked to do more than they are accustomed to. The magic word here is 'progressive' – each day you ask the muscles to do a little bit more work. The good news here is that the less physical activity you are accustomed to, the greater the potential for improvement.
- **Reversibility** Any improvements attained through exercise will disappear over a period of weeks if activity levels are not maintained. This is often referred to as the principle of 'use it or lose it'. This is precisely what happens to you in hospital after a heart attack.
- **Specificity** The improvements that you gain from any increased

activity will vary according to which muscles are used and how they are used. For example, tossing the caber will not improve your ability to run a half marathon or even to walk fast. This is because tossing the caber requires great power and strength in the arms whereas running and fast walking require stamina in the legs. Muscle strength, stamina, suppleness (flexibility) and motor skills (balance, coordination, etc.) are all components of fitness that can be improved with appropriate specifically selected activities.

What is progressive aerobic exercise?

Aerobic exercise uses oxygen to fuel the exercise. It should take place at a sustained level for at least five minutes, and should leave you feeling pleasantly breathless and a bit tired. Ideally, it should last for at least 20 minutes. If you are so exhausted by the end of it that you can barely speak, then you have done too much. High intensity exercise like lifting weights or running 100 metres (109 yards) flat-out is *anaerobic exercise* – it does not use oxygen – and is strongly to be discouraged if you are recovering from a heart attack.

Aerobic exercise uses large groups of muscles, e.g. in the legs and arms, in a continuous, dynamic and rhythmic manner. Walking is the most accessible exercise that most people can manage and is to be recommended in that it uses most of the muscles in the body. Jogging, cycling and swimming are also good forms of aerobic exercise, although if you were not used to doing them before your heart attack you would be advised not to try them until you are in phase 3 or 4 of the recovery period, i.e. when you are undertaking a rehabilitation programme or have completed one.

The other important feature of exercise that cannot be emphasised strongly enough is that it should be *progressive*. This can best be illustrated if you use an exercise bike. If, at a given load on the bike, you can pedal away for five minutes and then feel you've had enough – you're breathless and your heart's pounding – that's fine. The next day you should aim to pedal for six minutes, then for seven minutes the next day and eight minutes the day after and so on until you are up to, say, ten minutes. Perhaps to your surprise, you'll discover that while on the first day you were tired after five minutes, by the fifth day you can manage 10 minutes. Each day you will be able to manage a little more before your body says enough.

But that's not the end of it. Once you've got up to 10 minutes, put a slightly heavier load on the exercise bike for the next day's session.

Then you're back to five minutes pedalling before you've had enough. But the next day you can manage six minutes with the heavier load, then seven minutes the next day, and so on.

By gradually increasing the load and increasing the time on the bike, you will find that you will have pushed up your body's tolerance of exercise, perhaps to a level you hadn't thought possible for years. If you are walking, you can achieve the same effect by walking a bit faster each day, walking a bit further, walking up steeper or longer hills.

The important feature is that the exercise should be progressive. Each day, or each exercise session (perhaps they are every two or three days), you should aim to do a little bit more before you stop.

What do I gain from progressive aerobic exercise?

- Aerobic exercise increases the ability of the body to extract oxygen from the blood. Therefore the heart doesn't have to beat so fast to get the blood to the muscles – the muscles take more oxygen from each bit of blood that is pumped around them.

- Aerobic exercise increases the number of tiny blood vessels that carry the blood to the muscles – they form more branches and connections around the muscles. Therefore more blood is taken into the muscles and again the heart doesn't have to beat so fast.

- Aerobic exercise brings the blood pressure down, so that the heart doesn't have to work so hard pumping the blood around.

- Aerobic exercise increases the overall volume of blood in the body. At any one time, the blood is carrying more oxygen around simply because there is more of it.

- Aerobic exercise increases the amount of the chemical in the blood that carries the oxygen (haemoglobin or Hb). A unit of blood can therefore carry more oxygen around the body.

- All this extra ability to carry more oxygen in the blood and for the muscles to extract more oxygen from the blood means that the heart doesn't have to beat so fast when you undertake some exercise or activity. This allows more time for the heart to fill with blood each time it beats; it is stretched more and responds with a stronger pumping action.

These are a lot of benefits. What they mean in practical terms is that you have more stamina – you can do more before your heart complains. This reduces the chance of angina pain and the risk of a subsequent heart attack. This is an easy clearcut way to understand *primary gain* or benefit.

But there are also a number of *secondary gains* or benefits, i.e. changes that occur that have an indirect impact on the risk of a subsequent heart attack:

- Aerobic exercise brings down the overall cholesterol level in the blood. This reduces the risk of the arteries furring up and getting blocked, which in turn reduces the risk of angina and a heart attack. Indeed, some studies have shown that regular exercise can reduce the furring up of the arteries that has already occurred, i.e. can help make your coronary arteries healthier and remove some of the blockages that have built up over the years.
- Aerobic exercise reduces the stickiness of the blood. It is therefore less likely to form clots and to fur up the coronary arteries.
- Aerobic exercise increases the one form of cholesterol in the bloodstream that is good – HDL cholesterol. This also means that the risk of angina and heart attack is reduced.
- Aerobic exercise increases your lean muscle mass – very simply, you develop more muscle.
- Aerobic exercise reduces the amount of fat you carry around – it burns up fat rather than other body tissues. This will help you lose weight, so your heart doesn't have to work so hard providing the oxygen just to carry around the extra weight.
- Aerobic exercise will favourably alter the balance between blood glucose and insulin, reducing your risk of suffering from diabetes. As diabetes is a high risk factor for coronary heart disease, this is also going to have an impact on your risk of angina and another heart attack.
- As has already been explained, aerobic exercise reduces your blood pressure. High blood pressure is a risk factor for coronary heart disease, so this is also going to help reduce your risk of angina and heart attacks.
- Last, but by no means least, aerobic exercise makes you feel good. You feel healthier, you can do more without feeling pooped, you feel more in charge of your life, you feel more self-confident, you get a better image of yourself.

How do I know when I've had enough?
There are all sorts of ways of measuring the intensity of a given activity or exercise and of determining when you should stop. In theoretical terms, it is generally accepted that the most effective training intensity

for achieving aerobic fitness is between 50 and 70 per cent of your maximum capacity for effort. Maximum capacity is when you flog your guts out and end up collapsed on the ground gasping for air and unable to speak. If you are recovering from a heart attack, this is not a good state to be in. However, exercising to a level that is 50 to 70 per cent of your potential maximum level is a healthy target to be aimed for. But how do we measure this 50 to 70 per cent level?

First you can be hooked up to sophisticated machines that measure the amount of oxygen you are consuming. These are accurate, but are not portable and are not cheap. And they need a technician to operate them.

You can also use formulae based on your heart rate. There are various formulae available. The simplest assumes that the maximum heart rate (the number of times your heart beats per minute) that is reasonable is 220 minus your age. If you are 50 years old, then your maximum heart rate would be 220 - 50 = 170 beats per minute; if you are 75 years old, then your maximum is 220 - 75 = 145 beats per minute. If you are exercising to 50 to 70 per cent of this level, then your heart rate should be in the range 85 to 119 beats per minute if you are 50 years old, and 73 to 102 beats per minute if you are 75 years old.

But how do you measure your heart rate? There are gadgets that strap around your chest and give a readout on a wristwatch-type monitor. These are very accurate and reliable, but cost about £40 in 1995. An easier alternative is to learn to take your wrist pulse and count the number of beats per minute (or the number of beats in 30 seconds, then multiply by two). To take your wrist pulse, place the flats of the first two fingers of the right hand on the inside of your left wrist, two finger-widths below the wrist crease; you will feel a pulsing under your finger tips (you may need to move your fingers around slowly to locate the pulse). That is the wrist pulse; it is a blood vessel pulsing as the heart pumps. Look at a clock or watch with a second-hand and count the number of pulses in 30 seconds or a minute. Many people on cardiac rehabilitation programmes use this method of assessing their exercise levels and are very happy with it – it becomes a part of their life.

But not everyone is very good at measuring their own pulse. A bigger problem occurs with some of the drugs you might be on after a heart attack. Beta blockers in particular stabilise the heart rate and cause the heart to beat at an artificially low rate, whatever the exercise. This throws out the idea of calculating a formula for exercise levels based on your heart rate, for your heart rate is artificially low.

A much simpler method of assessing exercise levels is to use what is known as a *perceived exertion scale*, known as the *Borg scale* after the man who developed it. This is based on your own perception of the exertion involved in different exercise levels. It sounds very rough and approximate, but it is surprisingly accurate. In the following table a description of the level of exercise is given a rating on a scale:

Verbal description	Rating
Very very light – barely noticeable	0.5
Very light	1
Light	2
Moderate	3
Somewhat heavy	4
Heavy	5
	6
Very heavy	7
	8
	9
Very very heavy	10

Borg perceived exertion scale

The appropriate level of exertion to aim for is between 3 and 5 on this scale. To begin with you might need a little bit of guidance as to what the difference is between 3 (moderate) and 5 (heavy). If you are too cautious then you might underestimate what heavy exertion is – after heavy exertion you should be breathless and sweating but still capable of talking. If you are too determined, you might overdo it – if you are gasping for breath and can't speak, then you are up to 7 to 10. However, once you are clear about how you should feel at levels 3 to 5, you will find it very easy to use this system to assess any sort of exercise and there will be a close correlation between what you feel and your heart rate.

If you find this 10-point scale too complicated, there is an even simpler scale that rates your exercise level as:

- Too easy.
- Moderate.
- Too hard.

You should aim to exercise until you feel you are somewhere between moderate and too hard – too hard is when you are gasping for breath and can't talk.

Remember that for exercise to be of benefit:

- It has to go on for 20–30 minutes or longer.
- It has to make you slightly breathless at some stage – if it is a walk with a hill in the middle, say, then this breathless stage will occur during the walk and you may well have recovered your breath by the time you get home.
- It has to be progressive, so that you do a bit more each day until you reach a level of activity that you are comfortable with and that is doing some good – this should be 20–30 minutes at 3 to 5 on the Borg scale, at least three times a week.
- Once you have reached this level of activity you need to continue it for the rest of your life.

Pacing yourself

When you are set an exercise programme, or you devise a progressive activity programme of your own such as walking a bit further each day, you must make certain that you pace yourself. Not only does this mean doing a little more each day according to goals that have been set, either by the cardiac rehab team or by yourself, it also means not exceeding those goals, however good you might feel.

For example, a week after you come out of hospital you set yourself a goal of walking a quarter of a mile (or of a kilometre). You walk 200 yards down the road, then 200 yards (or metres) back to your house and you feel great – a bit breathless, your heart's thumping a bit, but after a couple of minutes you're fine and feeling really pleased with yourself. The next day, or in a couple of days' time, you can think about increasing your goal to 300 yards down the road and 300 yards back. What you must never do is, when you're in the middle of the 200 yards out and back, and feeling really on top of things, say to yourself' 'This is no trouble, I'll walk the extra 100 yards down to the corner.' You then have to walk the extra 100 yards back, you overdo it and when you get home you're knackered. What's more, you're frightened because your heart is really pounding and you don't know what to do the next day – more, less, the same, take a rest for a day? All because you exceeded your goal.

The message is, set a goal and stick to it. If it feels too much the first time you try it, set a slightly reduced goal the next day – do a bit less, maybe a couple of times round the garden instead of 200 yards down the road and back. If you achieve your goal easily, then increase the goal a bit the next day. But what you must not do – what will cause you and your body confusion – is forget about pacing yourself and deliberately ignore a goal you've set.

- Decide on your goals and stick to them.
- Amend future goals up or down *after* you've achieved one of your goals, not before.

But I don't want to be a fitness freak!

Some people who have had heart attacks take their exercise very seriously and go on to do marathons or take up some sport in a serious way. If this is what you want, fine – you will do yourself a lot of good.

But most people reading this book won't want to take things to that sort of extreme. They will want to live a healthy life, as free as possible from the risk of another heart attack and from the discomfort of angina. If that's what you want, then exercise and activity need to be incorporated into your life as part of your daily routine. There are all sorts of ways you can do this:

- For a start, use the car less and walk more, whether it's for shopping, taking the kids to school, going to the pub, going to work – where it's possible, walk.
- Use the stairs, not the lift, even if you've got to go up a few flights. As you get fitter, try trotting up the stairs.
- Try and fit a brisk walk into the daily routine – a mile or kilometre or two, so that you're out for half an hour. If you cannot manage this every day, try it two or three times during the week, with perhaps a longer walk – an hour or so – at the weekend.
- If you can afford it, get a bicycle and use that. With panniers you can go shopping on it.
- See what's going on at the local swimming pool. Most pools offer special sessions – before work, during the lunch hour, in the evening.
- See what's going on at the local leisure centre – badminton and short-mat bowls are just two activities that are suitable for you. Aerobics classes are ideal and most fitness centres can work out a programme for you that involves aerobic exercise on treadmills

or exercise bikes, with some strength and flexibility exercises worked in.

Walking a mile (1.6 km) at a brisk rate – so that it takes you about 20 minutes – uses 70 to 100 kilocalories of energy. This may not seem much when it takes 3,500 kilocalories to use up 1 lb (half a kilo) of fat – you'd need to walk 12 – 15 miles (20 – 5 km) to burn it off. But do some sums. That would mean about four to five hours of exercise, whether it's walking, cycling, swimming, playing badminton or mowing the lawn with a hand mower. If you spread that over the week – say a couple of miles brisk walk a day with a dog, then a five-mile (eight kilometre) walk at the weekend – you'd gain some huge benefits.

- You'd directly reduce your risk of a heart attack.
- There's a fair chance you'd start to remove the atheroma – the gunk that furs up your arteries – in your coronary arteries.
- If you ate no more than usual, you'd lose a pound (half a kilo) in weight each week.
- And you'd feel enormously better – fitter, happier, more relaxed, more content with life.

What you can expect

In this section we'll look at what you can expect in the way of formal exercise/rehabilitation programmes after your heart attack.

In hospital
Once upon a time, when you came into hospital after a heart attack you were kept in bed for weeks – it was thought the rest allowed your heart to heal. How wrong they were. It is now understood that this is the most harmful thing you can do – the body goes out of condition, the muscles waste away, the blood circulation stagnates and the whole healing process goes slow.

As has already been explained, your exercise programme gets going within hours of your arriving in hospital. In the first day you will be helped out of bed and into a chair for a while. This will seem like a huge effort. Remember the Borg perceived exertion scale? Getting out of bed will be well up to 5 on the scale, very hard. Then a bit later on you will be helped back into bed. Another effort of 5 on the Borg scale. After all that you'll probably have a snooze.

Later you may be helped out of bed for a wash while you're sat in a chair – again, it will probably seem like a major effort. You'll probably be left in the chair for a while afterwards, then helped back into bed. That will probably bring on another snooze.

Then a physiotherapist will come round to see you and talk to you about breathing exercises and exercises that you can do while still in bed. The breathing exercises will encourage deep breathing – as you breathe in put your hand on your tummy and try to push it out. This will take air down into the bottom of the lungs and ensure that sputum doesn't accumulate there. Deep breathing can be hard to learn to begin with – most people breathe with only the top part of their lungs, with only their shoulders moving. But as you learn to breathe by moving your tummy in and out it becomes very easy, almost second nature. And it has the great advantage that it relaxes you and calms you down – important to remember when you get tensed up and worried. A few seconds of deep breathing quickly relaxes you. If you can remember it, you should do some deep breathing every quarter of an hour when you are awake.

You may be encouraged to do some simple movements to keep your joints active and to give your muscles something to do:

- Move your fingers about for a minute or so every now and then, as if you're playing the piano.
- Hold out your arms and move your hands up and down from the wrist, then around in a circle from the wrist (if the drip tubes don't get in the way).
- Move your shoulders up and down and around, first one way then the other.
- Slowly turn your head from side to side and look over each shoulder if you can.
- Without raising your legs up, point your feet up and down, then circle them round, first one way then the other. This is a very important movement as it helps stop the blood stagnating in the feet.
- Tighten your thigh muscles for 5–10 seconds, then relax them. Repeat this five times.
- When you are sitting in a chair, bend your knees, then straighten them. Do this two or three times.

These movements will all help keep your joints supple and will help the blood circulation in the limbs. Try and do them for five minutes five times a day all the time you are in hospital and when you are sitting down and resting when you get home.

Within a day or two of coming into hospital you will be helped out of bed for a walk. It may only be a walk around the bed and you will certainly find it pretty tiring – maybe up to 5 on the Borg scale – but you'll be able to do it. Once you've done it once, ask if you can get out of bed and walk around unaccompanied. The nurse or physiotherapist might want you to take another accompanied walk before you can get up and walk on your own or they might be quite happy to let you do it alone. If you were pretty fit before your heart attack you should have little difficulty getting going again, but if you were unfit before your heart attack you will probably need to have an eye kept on you – making an effort is one thing, but doing too much is not so sensible at this stage.

The next day you will be sitting out for longer. You might have an accompanied walk down the ward, perhaps to the loo. If you feel you can manage this, ask for it. If not, make certain you walk round the bed and back when you have the energy. The day after you will be able to walk to the loo unaccompanied; a couple of times in the day might seem quite enough, but if you can manage more, do it.

Once you are allowed to wander around without supervision, gradually extend the range of your walks. You can walk around the ward, particularly if it is a racetrack-style ward. You can go down the corridor outside the ward, but always remember that you've got to come back as well. Ask before doing this – the staff might not want you out of their sight. When you have visitors, walk with them part of the way when they leave, although again check with the staff that this is all right. Not only will this show you how much you can do, but it will also make it clear to your spouse or partner or close family members that you are not an invalid and won't need to be wrapped in cotton-wool when you get home. You might even feel that you can cope with going to the hospital shop, but again ask before doing it. At some stage you will be accompanied up and down a flight of stairs, so that the staff can be sure you can cope with the stairs at home. This will really make you puff, but once you have done it once, ask if you can do it again on your own, unaccompanied, maybe later the same day or the next day.

For some heart attack patients the idea of walking through the hospital to the shop might seem like no great effort at all. For most it might seem like an insurmountable challenge. A lot will depend on your fitness level before the heart attack and the rest on determination.

You will recover – and the sooner you can get yourself going, the quicker this recovery will be – but don't be disheartened if you are making slower progress than the person in the next bed. They might have been fitter than you in the first place or not had so serious a heart attack. You will catch up later.

Going home

Before you go home the hospital staff will have ensured that:

- You can walk about on your own unaided.
- You can manage a flight of stairs.

If you can do this, then they will be happy that your activity levels are satisfactory for you to cope at home.

You might have also been given an exercise ECG test, which will have told the hospital staff quite a lot about the extent of the damage to your heart. Just as importantly, it will have shown you (and your spouse or partner, if they were present) just how much you can do, even at this early stage in your recovery. It will have really puffed you out, but you won't have been killed or collapsed by it. That is what your heart can stand up to, even at this early stage.

Remember that what you have been capable of doing during your last day or so in hospital, including your exercise ECG if you've had one, you will be perfectly capable of doing on your first day home. This is the activity level you can build on when you get home.

Before you go home you will undoubtedly be given a sheet or booklet by the rehabilitation nurse or physiotherapist outlining a progressive exercise programme for your first few weeks at home. This will be a very basic programme and will outline the bare minimum that you should be able to manage. Discuss with the nurse or physiotherapist what you can do in addition to what is on the sheet or in the booklet; if you show that you are determined to make an effort they will be able to give you lots of ideas.

Getting going again

When you are sent home from hospital, as just mentioned, you should have been given a sheet or booklet, produced by the hospital, giving you some guidance on what exercise you should be doing over the next few weeks. Some hospitals are much better than others in what they produce: in some cases you might only get a single sheet of paper with some vague guidance on what you should be doing; in others you might get a booklet with specific strength and flexibility exercises detailed in them plus some firm guidelines on a progressive walking programme that gradually builds up your stamina. In some cases, regrettably, you will get nothing. The last section in this chapter gives some specific suggestions regarding exercise programmes over these first few weeks out of hospital. Here we will merely discuss what you ought to be doing in general terms:

- If you have been given specific ideas on exercise by the hospital, make certain you do them every day, or whenever advised, and make certain you do a little more each day.
- If you have only been given vague ideas by the hospital, try and work out how you can best put them into practice in your home. Consult the detailed suggestions on exercise at the end of this chapter for more ideas if you want them.
- If you have received very little guidance and advice, make use of the ideas in this book on a regular daily basis.
- If you do nothing else, walk.
- Very simply, you should be doing more each day.

On your first day after you come home from hospital you should be able to manage somewhere between 5 and 15 minutes walking. If you are nervous of going out so soon, walk around the house, perhaps going up and down stairs once. If you have a garden, make use of it.

If you are happy about walking outside at this stage, you should warm up your system in the house first – pace up and down the hall or the largest room for a minute or so before going out. If it is cold, wrap up well – cold weather tends to make heart attack patients feel weaker and brings on angina sooner.

To begin with try walking around the block or just walk down to the corner and back. It will probably seem like hard work, but shouldn't leave you so breathless that you can't speak. Read the section on the Borg scale earlier in this chapter so that you know about which level you should take yourself to – you should feel as if you've made a moderate to hard effort, you should be sweating, you should be puffing a bit and you should be aware of your heart beating faster than usual.

If it takes you longer than 10 minutes to recover, you have done too much. Don't give up. Repeat the walk the next day, but don't go so far or don't go so fast. If you get chest pains during the walk, stop and take a nitrate tablet or spray (see page 49), then continue when you are comfortable.

If you have no after-effects after the walk – you're not puffing, you don't feel as if you've made any real effort, you're not aware of your heart beating harder or faster – then you are fitter than you think. The next day walk a bit further, or a bit faster, until you do feel as if you are up to 4 or 5 on the Borg scale. You should be breathing harder than usual, you should be aware of your heart beating harder and faster, you should be sweating slightly and you should feel as if you've made an effort, but everything should return to normal after one to five minutes. Don't be afraid of any of these feelings. They won't kill you, they are merely an indication that the body has made an effort. Tomorrow or the next day you will be able to do the same thing without so much effort, as the body will be that bit fitter. If you don't make this effort, the body will stay the same, unfit and unhealthy, and your risk of another heart attack will not be reduced. To reduce that risk you need to make an effort with your exercising.

This also goes for work around the house. Just because you've had a heart attack doesn't mean you can give up on all the chores around the house and garden that you used to do. You will undoubtedly need to ease yourself back into the routine gently – you will get tired and will need to rest and have a nap every now and then. But you are not an invalid and shouldn't see yourself as one – nor should you let other people see you as one. The important thing is to do a bit more each day, whether it's exercises, walking, chores around the house or the gardening.

By about five weeks after your heart attack the heart will have finished its repair work. Scar tissue will have formed where the heart muscle was damaged by the interruption to the blood supply. The nearby sections of heart muscle will have strengthened and nearby blood vessels will have developed to compensate for the area of muscle affected by the blocked artery. This means that your exercise programme can become more vigorous and is why cardiac rehab programmes don't start until at least six weeks after the heart attack.

Rehabilitation programmes

If there is a local cardiac rehabilitation programme, whether it is run by the hospital, by the local GPs or the local leisure centre, you should be offered a place on it somewhere between the third and eighth week after your heart attack. At all costs you should take this place up, however much it might be a problem getting to and from the sessions or finding the time to spend on the course. As much as anything else you can do, a structured rehabilitation course will help you get back to leading a normal life, and one that is probably healthier and more active than the life you led before your heart attack.

One of the key ingredients of a properly managed cardiac rehabilitation programme is that your fitness and activity levels will be accurately assessed and then closely monitored throughout the programme. You will be encouraged to undertake tougher exercise programmes than you might otherwise do on your own, but it will be in a safe and monitored environment, with staff on hand to deal with any emergencies that might occur.

- To begin with you should have an exercise ECG test before you even start the programme. This is so that the staff can assess what your level of fitness and activity is, and design a programme for you that will be within your capabilities.
- Once you are on the programme you will be monitored for your heart rate (the number of times it beats per minute), your blood pressure and your exertion level, perhaps using the Borg scale. Not only will the staff carry out this monitoring, but they will probably teach you how to carry it out yourself. This will be great for your self-confidence, as you will feel more in control of what you're doing.
- You will be in a group of other heart attack patients, some of whom will be starting the programme at the same time as you and some of whom will be midway through or at the end of the programme. Just by observing what other people are doing, you will be able to assess what you should be, and can expect to be, doing while you are on the programme.
- On some rehab programmes spouses or partners are involved at various stages. This allows them to see what you are capable of doing (it might come as a shock to them), and will enable them to encourage you and support you in the exercise you are taking outside the programme.

In a rehabilitation programme, the emphasis will be on aerobic as opposed to anaerobic exercise, as explained at the beginning of this chapter: Also:

- You will be taught about warm-up and wind-down exercises at the beginning and end of each session. These are very important and you should remember them when you are exercising at home.

- You will be given exercises to build up your stamina, perhaps on an exercise bike or a treadmill, or walking around the hospital grounds, or stepping up and down onto a bench or a step.
- You will be given exercises to build up the strength in your legs and arms and other parts of your body.
- You will be given exercises to make you more flexible – stretching exercises and bending and twisting movements.
- You may be taught breathing exercises.
- You will be given a relaxation session at each class, and taught how to relax and to deal with stress without getting wound up.

The size of the rehab team will vary from centre to centre, depending on the availability of staff and the resources (including money) that are made available. At the very least there will be a cardiac/coronary care nurse and a physiotherapist; in some centres, that's all there is. At most centres, though, some or all of the following will be part of the team; they may not all be present all of the time – some may only come in for part of the sessions or just for specific sessions:

- The programme will probably be run by a cardiac/coronary care nurse – someone who has specialised in coronary care and who has worked in the CCU and on the cardiology ward. They will be responsible for the routine monitoring that goes on in the sessions – heart rate and blood pressure, for example.
- There will be at least one physiotherapist, who will be supervising the exercise programmes and advising you on what you can do, how best to do it, what equipment to use and what benefits you are gaining.
- There may be an exercise physiologist, although this is rare. An exercise physiologist's training overlaps with that of a sports trainer, a physiotherapist and a nurse, so they are ideally qualified for a cardiac rehab programme. There are not many of them around at the moment, though.
- A dietitian will be able to advise you and your spouse or partner on what sorts of foods you should be eating regularly. If you have a weight problem, they will be able to help in reducing it.
- The pharmacist will talk to you about the various drugs you might be on after a heart attack, discuss any problems you might

have with side-effects and perhaps recommend changes to specific drugs or dosages that might suit you better.

- After a heart attack there are many psychological consequences, ranging from fear and anger through grief and depression to acceptance or, in some cases, denial. A clinical psychologist often attends the rehab sessions to talk about these consequences and to discuss any problem areas with you. Often it is a relief to find out that these psychological consequences are perfectly normal and to talk to someone about how to deal with them.

- Some rehab programmes make use of a massage therapist. This might sound a bit odd at first, but they can provide a tremendously useful service if your joints are stiff or aching. They are also very good at teaching relaxation techniques – very useful for dealing with stress.

Most cardiac rehabilitation programmes will be hospital-based, making use of the physiotherapy gym and perhaps an ancillary room. You therefore go to the hospital for the rehab sessions. Some schemes, though, are run by GPs, in which case the sessions might be anywhere – in the health centre, in the local leisure centre, even in the village hall. This may well make the programme easier to get to than a district hospital. There are a few schemes run by local leisure/sports centres or by private fitness centres; they invariably work with a local GP or a doctor who provides the assessment and monitoring that is essential to such a scheme.

Cardiac rehab programmes usually provide a series of sessions that run for between 6 and 12 weeks, and once you have attended your quota of classes that's that – you're fit and well and on your own. A few of the larger rehab schemes do provide longer programmes, but these are rare.

At the end of a rehab programme you should be well aware of what precipitated your heart attack in the first place – probably a mixture of smoking, diet and inactivity. You should also be clear about what you need to do to reduce the risk not only of suffering another heart attack but also of suffering from further symptoms of coronary heart disease. What you do with the advice and guidance you have received is up to you, but you should understand that with some relatively simple and straightforward changes to your life you will be able to lead a much fitter and happier life, considerably clearer of the risk of a heart attack than you were.

Long term

In the long term, therefore, you need to build on the lessons you have learned in hospital, in the period after you left hospital and while you were on the cardiac rehab programme:

- First and foremost, if you are a smoker you need to give up smoking permanently. This can be a big problem for some people and will be examined in more detail later in the book.
- You need to take regular exercise, primarily to keep up your stamina but also to keep up the levels of strength and flexibility you should have developed on the rehab programme. This exercise should be an activity that you enjoy and that you can happily spend some time on each week, whether it is walking, swimming, cycling, some sport, active work in the garden or a combination of all of these things. This is something that should never leave you.
- You need to give some thought to the food you eat. Again, this can seem like a problem for some people and is dealt with in more detail later in the book.

Taking these ideas on board and implementing them in the short term may seem no problem – indeed, for some it might seem quite exciting as they take their life in hand and turn it round. But in the long term there might be the fear that these changes won't stick. One source of support can be to join some sort of group of people who have had heart attacks or who have suffered or suffer from the symptoms of coronary heart disease. There are various sorts of groups around:

- Self-help groups are what they say they are – groups of people who have had heart attacks or who are married to or live with people who have had attacks, who gather together regularly to compare notes and ideas, organise social events, visit people or families who have just suffered a heart attack, or just get together to talk. Such groups might be organised by someone at the health centre or they might be outside the health service completely. Ask at your health centre or local library if there is such a group in your area.
- Heartbeat groups are groups that fall under the umbrella of the British Heart Foundation. The BHF can help set up a group and then will keep it supplied with newsletters, information, etc., plus providing links with the national network of Heartbeat groups. Your health centre or the cardiac clinic will be able to let you know if

there is a Heartbeat group in your area; alternatively you can contact the BHF direct (their address is at the end of the book).
- Some rehabilitation programmes run their own 'graduate' groups. These might offer the opportunity of a long-term structured exercise programme, but in general they tend to be self-help 'talking shops' where you can get together with other people in a similar situation to you and swap notes, socialise, support each other and keep in touch.

The support such groups can offer can be very valuable – if you are still exercising, off smoking and eating sensibly a year after your heart attack you stand a very good chance of keeping up this pattern in the long term, and the support of a self-help group can be very important.

Perhaps the one slight criticism of such groups is that they can tend to foster the image of the heart attack patient as someone different from the rest of society. If you have had a heart attack, for a while you *are* different – you are ill. Then you are recovering. Then you are well again. To be sure, some people who have heart attacks have hearts that are so damaged that they are limited in what they can do for the rest of their lives. However, most people can recover from a heart attack and lead the same or a healthier, more active life than they enjoyed before the heart attack. Being a member of a group of people who have all had heart disease or a heart attack can be a great support – indeed, you can be a great support to other people – but try not to think of yourself as someone who is in some way incapacitated by what has happened.

What you can do yourself

If you are unfortunate to live in an area that does not seem to have a cardiac rehab programme and you have a heart attack, what do you do? Or maybe you have a heart attack on holiday and are rushed into the local district hospital, then sent home to a nearby relative while you gain the strength to be driven back to your own home. You are then likely to fall down a gap between the two rehab programmes and end up with nothing. This section looks at what you can do yourself to try and fill the gap, and, if all else fails, outlines an exercise rehabilitation programme that you can use at home.

Encourage provision by others
If no one has approached you about a rehabilitation programme by the

time you are out of the CCU and on to the general cardiology ward, ask your nurse why not. It might be a genuine oversight. If you are in a hospital away from your normal area, they might not be bothering with you because they think you will get on to a rehab programme when you get home. Tell them you want to get as much help from the rehab team as you can while you are in hospital, even if you aren't going to be on their programme later – don't turn down any help or information.

If there is no rehabilitation programme, ask the doctors on their ward round why not. Obviously a rehab programme won't be set up specially for you, but it might push them into thinking about setting one up in the future. And it might prompt them to give you more help and advice than you would otherwise have got.

As soon as you get home and see your GP, ask them what is available locally in the way of a cardiac rehabilitation programme. They might be linked to or know of a GP-run or a GP-referral scheme nearby. Tell them that you want to get onto such a scheme.

If all these enquiries draw a blank, contact the British Heart Foundation. They keep a register of all the cardiac rehabilitation programmes around the country and will be able to let you know of nearby schemes. Armed with this information, go back to your GP or cardiac clinic and find out how you can get onto one of these programmes.

Another option is to visit your local leisure or fitness centre and ask what is available. If they say they do have a rehab programme, ask them if a GP or doctor carries out the initial assessment of heart attack patients (the answer should be 'Yes'). Would you be put through an exercise ECG before being accepted (again the answer should be 'Yes'). Do they have heart rate and blood pressure monitoring equipment (again, they should answer 'Yes'). And does the person running the course have the RSA-Sports Council 80-hour Exercise to Music certificate (this should be the bare minimum)? If most of the answers to these questions are 'No', then they are not offering a programme that would be safe for you at this stage. If they are interested in offering such a course (and they may well be if you tell them that nothing else is available in your area), tell them to get in touch with the British Association for Cardiac Rehabilitation, who will be able to offer them guidance on setting one up.

The Heart Manual

In Scotland many people do not live close to their district hospital.

Scotland also has the worst record in the world for coronary heart disease – a lot of people have heart attacks in Scotland. There is therefore a great need for cardiac rehabilitation, while at the same time it is hard or impossible for people from many areas of the country to attend a programme that is run in a district hospital.

A group in Edinburgh have therefore developed something called *The Heart Manual*. This is a 120-page self-help manual, plus a relaxation tape and an explanatory tape, that details a six-week programme of cardiac rehabilitation – and it works.

You can't buy it over the counter in your local bookshop, though. You can only get it if someone at the cardiac clinic or at your health centre goes on a two-day training course in Edinburgh. They can then act as a local facilitator and explain to users of *The Heart Manual* exactly how it should be used properly. *The Heart Manual* is not a book you can just pick up and dive into, and you can only obtain it via a trained facilitator.

If there is no cardiac rehabilitation programme available in your area, you could explain to your cardiac clinic or your GP what *The Heart Manual* is (a self-administered cardiac rehabilitation programme), how to find out about it (the address is at the back of this book), that it needs a local facilitator (trained for two days in Edinburgh) and that you would like to make use of it. Would they therefore consider sending someone off on the facilitator's training course? You could also tell them that *The Heart Manual* has been designed 'to allow any general hospital or health centre to deliver post-heart attack rehabilitation with the minimum of disruption and cost and with little or no demand on existing infrastructures and staffing levels'. No one is going to say 'Yes' just because you ask them these questions, but if they say 'No' you can always ask 'Why?' And if it improves your chances of receiving cardiac rehabilitation, the effort on your part has to be worth it.

Self-help

What follows is an outline exercise programme you can use at home if no form of organised cardiac rehabilitation programme is available. This chapter has already given various ideas and suggestions that you can use at home; this section gives specific ideas. Two points must be understood, though:

- Reference is made to the Borg scale, detailed earlier in this chapter.

If you are going to exercise at home with no support from a formal rehabilitation programme, you need to understand this scale. On the one hand, the exercises need to make you feel you've done something; on the other hand, you should not overdo things so that you are so breathless you cannot speak.

• If you start to feel chest pain or any other angina symptoms when you are exercising, use your GTN/nitrate tablets or spray, take a break until the symptoms have gone (if necessary take another tablet or dose of spray), then start again.

So that you can keep yourself well-motivated and see how well you are progressing, buy a desk diary – one with plenty of space for each day – and write down exactly what you do every day. One suggestion is, for each day, give details of:

• The strength and flexibility exercises – how many, how long, how many sequences, rating on the Borg scale.
• Walking – how far, how much time it took, hills, rating on the Borg scale.
• Other aerobic exercise, e.g. swimming, cycling – what the activity is, how much time, rating on the Borg scale.
• Other daily activities, e.g. cooking, washing up, hoovering, shopping, gardening, mowing the lawn – what the activity is, how much time, rating on the Borg scale.
• Keep this diary going, even in an abbreviated form, for at least a year after you leave hospital.

Remember that one of the most important pieces of advice this book gives is that if you want to reduce the risk of another heart attack you have to make permanent lifelong changes to your life. This includes taking more exercise on a regular basis. Long after your heart attack has receded into the past, check out your exercise and activity diary and see what you were doing six weeks or 12 weeks after leaving hospital. Are you still doing that amount of activity? If you are – or you are doing more – all well and good. But if you are not, then perhaps you need to go back to your diary and start again on what you began when you left hospital.

Strength and mobility exercises
These exercises can be carried out in the smallest home – even in a flat.

They require next to no equipment, but you might need some help to begin with:

- When you first start, if possible get someone to read out the instructions to you so that you aren't stopping every now and then to read them yourself. After a while you will get to know them by heart.
- Get someone to count/time the exercises as well, if necessary.

Activity	How long/many	How to do it
March on the spot	30 secs–1 min	March on the spot, lifting the knees up. Keep the back straight and hold the stomach in. The arms should swing in time with the steps.
Arm raises	30 secs	Stand with your feet hip-width apart, arms by your side. Lift your arms slowly up to shoulder level, then slowly lower them again. If you can't lift to shoulder level, lift them as high as you can, but try and lift them a little higher the next day. Lift one arm at a time if necessary.
Step ups	30 secs–1 min	Use the bottom step of you stairs, or a solid wooden box if you live in a bungalow or flat. Step up and down, changing the foot you step up with every 10 seconds. Use a handrail/chairback for support if necessary.
Wall push-ups	8–12	Face the wall at arm's length, feet hip-width apart. Raise your arms and place your hands on the wall. Lean against the wall, then bend your arms, keeping your body

		straight. Bend your arms until your nose touches the wall, then straighten your arms until you are back at the starting position. Try to keep your back straight all the time – don't arch it.
Sit and stand	30 secs–1 min	Sit on the edge of an upright chair, feet slightly apart, arms crossed on your chest. Stand up, then sit down again. Try not to lean forward – it should be your legs that are doing all the work.
Bicep curls	8–12	Get two tins of baked beans, or something similar, and hold them, one in each hand. Stand up straight, with the arms by the sides, fingers facing forwards. Bend the arm at the elbow so that the fingers (and tins) touch the front of the shoulders. Return to the starting position.

A single sequence of strength/flexibility exercises

- When you have finished one complete sequence (the whole chart), go back and repeat it twice, so that you do three sequences in total.
- As you get fitter you can put more effort into the exercises: step higher, raise the arms more slowly, do the wall push-ups more slowly, sit and stand more slowly, do the bicep curls more slowly.
- If you want to, buy some dumb-bells (available at most sports shops) and use them instead of the tins of beans for the bicep curls. Don't get dumb-bells that are too heavy to begin with.
- As you get fitter you can also increase the length of time/number of each activity.
- When you feel up to it, add on an extra sequence.
- Always keep to a limit of 3–5 on the Borg scale.

- It will be very valuable to you to keep a daily record of what you do – how long you do each activity, how many times, where you think you got to on the Borg scale. You will then be able to see how much you are progressing and how much you achieve over the weeks.

Walking
The following ideas on a progressive walking programme should be looked upon as an average. If you were very unfit before your heart attack or have suffered a lot of damage to the heart muscle, you may not be able to manage as much as is outlined in the time given. Do not worry, just take more weeks to get up to the targets. On the other hand, if you were fit before your heart attack, you may find that this programme does not take you to 3–5 on the Borg scale, in which case you can move up to longer distances in a shorter time. The important point to remember is that each session of walking should take you to the level on the Borg scale given in the table.

Week after leaving hospital	Duration (minutes)	Distance per day	Frequency	Level on Borg scale
1	5	200 yds/182 metres	1–2	2–3
2	10	¼ mile/¼ km	2	2–3
3	15	½ mile/½ km	2	2–3
4	20	¾ mile/¾ km	1–2	3–5
5	25–30	1 mile/1½ km	1–2	3–5
6	30–40	1–2 miles/1½–3 km	1–2	3–5
Thereafter	30–40	1½–2 miles/2–3 km	1–2	3–5

Walking guidelines for heart attack patients

- Always walk at a pace that feels comfortable but that is not too slow.
- Warm up and warm down by starting and finishing your walk at a slower pace.
- Keep a diary of your walking – how far, how much time, what you felt like.
- If you feel tired for some time after completing a walk, reduce the distance or the speed the next day.

- Do not walk for 30 – 40 minutes after a main meal.
- If you get a chest pain or any other angina symptoms, use your GTN/nitrate tablets or spray, wait until the symptoms go, then continue your walk at a reduced pace.
- Incorporate these walks into the daily routine where possible, so that they become part of your life. They could include a walk to the shops, or walking the dog – borrow a neighbour's dog if necessary or seriously think about getting one yourself.
- To begin with, avoid walking in extremes of weather – very cold and windy or very hot and humid.

Other activities
Walking is the ideal basis for exercise – it exercises a lot of muscles, everyone can do it and you don't need any special clothes or kit. However, other activities could be incorporated into your life to give more variety.

- Swimming is very good, but unless you have done a lot of swimming before your heart attack it is probably best to wait until six weeks after leaving hospital before starting to swim lengths.
- Cycling can be on a real bicycle, but if you don't fancy that then maybe an exercise bike would be more suitable – you can use it on rainy or cold days and listen to music or watch the TV at the same time.
- Rowing machines are as adaptable as exercise bikes, but remember that they work both the upper and lower body at the same time. To begin with they will take you up to 3 – 5 on the Borg scale much faster than walking. Do not overdo it.

To give you a comparison of different activities, the accompanying table shows how many kilocalories you burn off, depending on what weight you are. It also gives one or two more ideas for activities.

Activity	Body weight			
	9 stone/ 56 kg	10 stone/ 62 kg	11 stone/ 68 kg	12 stone/ 75 kg
Cycling at 5 mph	36	40	44	47
Cycling at 10 mph	56	62	68	75
Walking at 3 mph	45	50	54	60
Swimming breast-stroke	91	100	110	121
Treading water	35	38	42	47
Dancing, ballroom	29	32	35	39
Dancing, aerobic	94	104	114	125

Kilocalories used up by different activities over 10 minutes

Finally

It cannot be emphasised enough that exercise is one of the keys to recovery from a heart attack and to minimising the risk of a recurrence. The following are the most important general points to be made in this chapter; you should understand them and be prepared to act on them.

- Listen to all the advice you receive on exercise and activity. Ask questions if you don't understand.
- Act on this advice as soon as you can, whether it's one day after your heart attack or 10 years after.
- If a cardiac rehabilitation programme is available to you, move heaven and earth to get onto it.
- If a cardiac rehabilitation programme is not available, find out where the nearest one is based and try your hardest to get onto that. (If you feel strong enough, let the cardiac unit that has been treating you know that they are letting you down by not providing a rehab progamme.)
- Incorporate the advice on exercise and activity into your daily life. You will be fitter, healthier, less stressed and happier. You will also be less at risk of a subsequent heart attack.
- Understand that exercise and activity should become part of your everyday life for the rest of your life.

8 Smoking

This could be the shortest chapter in the book, consisting of just two statements:

- Smoking kills you.
- Don't smoke.

Unfortunately life is far more complex than that. Most people know that smoking kills, although few realise quite how many health problems are due to it. And if you do smoke, it can be very difficult to give up – smoking is addictive, more addictive than heroin, and to quit smoking and stay a non-smoker is a major achievement.

If you have been in hospital after a heart attack, you will have been forced not to smoke for a few days. All hospitals are non-smoking zones now and the only places you can smoke are usually a long way from your bed. The one thing you can't do immediately after a heart attack is walk very far, so you will have become an enforced non-smoker. Build on this opportunity and remain a non-smoker if you can; this chapter suggests all sorts of strategies for keeping off cigarettes. And if you've gone back to smoking after you've left hospital, this chapter helps to explain why smoking is such a problem and what can be done to help you stop it.

The most important point to remember is that giving up smoking, however many attempts you have to make, is the most valuable thing you can do to reduce your risk of another heart attack.

The health risks

Tobacco contains a lot of different poisons, and we don't know the effect on the body of half of them yet. However, there are two that we know a lot about:

- **Carbon monoxide** This is the poisonous gas produced in car exhausts that people inhale when they commit suicide by running the engine in a closed garage or by connecting a hosepipe to the exhaust then running it in through the car window. Carbon monoxide is present in large quantities in cigarette smoke. It blocks the uptake of oxygen by the blood, then is carried around in the bloodstream to the cells; it can then kill the cells.

- **Nicotine** Nicotine has a whole collection of nasty effects: it damages the blood cells; it makes the blood clot more easily; it makes the blood vessel walls more liable to damage. All this increases the risk of blood clots forming and blocking the blood vessels. It also excites the heart, making it work harder and raising the blood pressure.

The harmful effects of smoking are usually accepted by the general population – smoking is the single most important cause of premature death, i.e. early death, in this country. But do you really realise how many diseases are caused by or aggravated by smoking? Let's look at coronary heart disease to begin with:

- Smoking accounts for nearly 20 per cent of all deaths from coronary heart disease.
- Smoking increases the risk of coronary heart disease by two to three times – the more you smoke, the greater the risk.

The damage to and blockage of blood vessels associated with smoking can cause other problems:

- The risk of a stroke (damage to the brain from a clot blocking a blood vessel in the brain) is doubled, even in young people.
- The risk of death from a stroke goes up by over 10 per cent.
- The risk of a sub-arachnoid haemorrhage (a bleed under the surface of the skull that then presses on the brain) is increased six-fold.
- Circulation is damaged in other parts of the body, leading to gangrene and amputation of the limbs.

Smoking causes lung cancer – most people know that. But it also causes lots of other cancers:

- It causes cancer in the breathing tubes.
- It causes cancer of the larynx – the voice box.
- It causes cancer of the mouth.
- It causes cancer of the oesophagus – the gullet.

- It also plays a part in cancers of the stomach, kidneys and bladder.

What else?

- It obviously causes diseases of the breathing system – bronchitis, catarrh, sinusitis, fluid on the lungs.
- It can cause duodenal ulcers – ulcers of the small intestine.
- It can cause dental decay.

Then there are other problems that are harder to define:

- Your senses of taste and smell are severely compromised.
- Your ability to take exercise is limited because you get breathless quickly.
- You smell like an ashtray.
- It costs you, and therefore your family, a lot of money.
- The diseases caused by passive smoking – inhaling other people's cigarette smoke – are a fact, although the risks are a matter for discussion. Whatever the discussion, the risks are real.
- Non-smokers don't like a smoke-filled atmosphere – it's an anti-social activity.
- Smokers and smoking cause 25 per cent of fires in the home.

Given all these problems, risks and diseases, it's perhaps a wonder anyone ever starts smoking. But, unfortunately, lots of people do, particularly young people and women, due to peer group pressure – 'All me mates smoke, so I started too' – and the effectiveness of tobacco advertising and marketing. And once you're hooked, it's very difficult to give up.

The benefits of smoking

There are none.

Every now and then a report or study surfaces that links smoking with alleviation of symptoms in such and such a disease – ulcerative colitis and Alzheimer's disease are two recent examples. But these reports and studies are invariably ambiguous in their conclusions, and even if the claimed benefits (usually slight) are true, they in no way counteract the risks and dangers that we have already listed.

'But what about my Uncle George? He smoked 60 cigarettes a day and lived to 92, when he was run over by a brewery delivery van when he was going into the pub.'

Everyone's got some sort of story like this and the explanation comes down to percentage chances of risk. If you smoke, your risk of coronary heart disease (and all sorts of other diseases) goes up, and each extra year you smoke the risk gets greater and greater. If you take 100 people like Uncle George, let's say that 99 will probably die of coronary heart disease or some other smoking-related disease. Uncle George was lucky; he was the 1 in 100 who didn't die of a smoking-related disease – although if the brewery van hadn't hit him he could well have died of a heart attack the next day.

If you smoke, you play Russian roulette. The more you smoke and the longer you smoke, the fewer blank bullets and the more live rounds there are in the pistol that you hold to your head.

How to give up

If you are a smoker and you're reading this book you already know that you should give up smoking. If you've read this chapter so far, then you probably want to give up. So you're already part way down the road to success.

Giving up smoking is not easy. You will probably try it a number of times. Each time you try it's a mark of success – you've wanted to give up so much you've actually tried it. Each time you go back to smoking it's a disappointment, but it's not a failure – you can try again. Very, very few people give up smoking on the first attempt and each time they go back to smoking it's not a failure, it's a delay. The hardest part is telling yourself that you want to give up – and then believing it.

There are three questions to consider if you are a smoker:

- What do you understand about the effect of smoking on your health? If you are unclear, reread the first part of this chapter. Go to your health centre and ask what information they can give you. Ask at the cardiac clinic about why you should give it up. You'll be inundated with information. Read it, watch it, listen to it and ask questions if you don't understand.
- Are you ready to give up smoking? You may want to give up – that means you are already part way down the road to stopping. But are you ready to give up? This is where you make the choice.
- What are your reasons for wanting to stop? Think about them, write

them down, pin them up where you can see them every day. You have made a choice and these are the reasons for your choice. They are very important. They might be the health benefits. They might be the social benefits. They might be financial benefits. They might be the fitness benefits. They might be all of these.

If you have answered all these questions, then you are a long way down the road to stopping. The rest of the journey will be a lot slower, but you've already travelled a great distance.

Three stages are now involved in giving up smoking and staying off smoking.

- You need to prepare yourself to give up smoking. This may not take long.
- You need to stop. This might take a number of attempts.
- You need to stay stopped. This may take some thought and organisation to begin with.

Preparing to stop

It is easy to think of all the nasty things that smoking does to you and then to say that if you stop you will avoid these nasties. This is fine.

But it is often more helpful and encouraging to think of the benefits that come with not smoking.

- My risk of another heart attack immediately starts to go down.
- Each day I stay off cigarettes my risk of another heart attack goes down further.
- I'll be able to breathe more easily.
- I'll lose that persistent cough.
- My food will become more tasty.
- I'll be able to smell things again.
- Other people won't think I'm smelly.
- When I kiss my children/grandchildren they won't think I smell like an ashtray.
- I'll find it easier to take up the exercise that is recommended for me.
- I'll save a fortune – hundreds of pounds a year.

Copy this list if you like. See if you can add to it. Talk about it with your partner or spouse or your family and see if they can add to it.

Side-effect	Cause	Coping
Craving	This is caused by the intense desire to smoke that is part of the addiction.	Distract yourself, e.g. with deep breathing. The craving gets less over the first months, and then goes.
Mood swings, irritability	You have lost an old friend – smoking/cigarettes. These symptoms are part of loss and grief.	You will come to accept this loss.
Coughing	This gets worse initially as your lungs clear out the effects of smoking.	It then gets better, then goes.
Moments of dizziness	More oxygen is getting to the body and brain.	The moments pass quickly and are not dangerous.
Feeling hungry	This can be intense.	Try not to eat sweets; fruit is better. The feelings subside over the weeks.
Constipation or diarrhoea	Your body is adjusting to life without an addictive drug.	This settles over the first couple of weeks.
Sleep problems	Again, this is adjustment to life without addiction.	And again, it settles over the first couple of weeks.

Possible withdrawal symptoms after giving up smoking

Over a week, keep a diary and log all the times, places and events when you have a cigarette. See if you can work out why you have a cigarette at a particular time or place. Then think about what you can do instead, after you've given up smoking. This might be difficult, but give it some thought and discuss it with other people.

It is important to involve other people, as they can give you support and help you over the difficult bits. The more people you tell you are going to give up smoking, the more people will be available to help you. Explain to them why you want to give up. Ask them for help.

Find out about relaxation techniques (see next chapter) to help you get over moments of tension when you would normally have a cigarette. A few deep relaxed breaths, or shrugging your shoulders up and then relaxing them a few times, is often all that is needed.

See if a friend or a member of the family wants to give up at the same time as you. If so, you can work together and help each other along, giving each other support at difficult times.

You should be undertaking an exercise programme as part of your cardiac rehab. Look upon this and giving up smoking as linked together in building a new fitter you.

You have to be aware that there will be side-effects once you stop smoking. You are probably aware that you might become irritable for a few days, but there are other possible effects as well. All these settle after a week or two. They are all withdrawal symptoms – after all, you are giving up an addiction.

The last stage of preparation for giving up smoking is to decide on a day and to think of it as your 'Quit Smoking Day'. It might be tomorrow, it might be next Monday or it might be a Saturday so you've got the weekend to adjust to the idea before going back to work. Stopping completely is a far more successful strategy than gradual reduction.

Stopping smoking
When you have got to your 'Quit Smoking Day' there are a number of things you can do to underline your decision.

- You can throw away all the bits and bobs that are involved with smoking. Throw away the cigarettes. Get rid of your matches. Get rid of your cigarette lighter – if it is particularly valuable to you, give it to someone else, preferably outside the household, and ask them to hold on to it for you for a year. Get rid of the ashtrays. If you smoke rollies, get rid of the papers and the tin and the tobacco and all the rest of the kit.
- Organise some sort of special activity to take your mind off the lack of cigarettes – go and visit the family, take the grandchildren to the zoo, go and visit the nearby stately home or gardens, go to a football match.
- Plan some sort of reward at the end of the day if you get through it without a cigarette – maybe a meal out or a bottle of wine. If it's your husband or wife or partner who's giving up, get them a little present.

Staying off the cigarettes

You've got through the first day without a cigarette. Now comes another hard bit – remaining a non-smoker. Some days will be easy and others may seem like no fun at all. Be aware of the fact that you will have bad days, days of temptation, especially at the beginning, and devise strategies for coping with them.

- Right from the beginning, think of yourself as a non-smoker. You are not someone who is giving up smoking, you are a non-smoker and have been a non-smoker from the moment you woke up on your 'Quit Smoking Day'.
- Each day you keep off cigarettes think of it as another success. If a day seems like a long time at the beginning, think in terms of morning, afternoon and evening, or even take each hour at a time.
- Try to avoid situations where other people smoke and are likely to offer you a cigarette, or you are likely to be tempted. Pubs are perhaps the worst places for temptation.
- Always go to non-smoking areas – in restaurants, buses, trains, cinemas, everywhere where they are available. If you've not used them before you'll be quite surprised how much more congenial they are – no smell, cleaner, tidier, no burn-holes in the carpet.
- Use your exercise programme as a diversion for the desire for a cigarette. This will not only give you something else to do instead of thinking of a cigarette, it will reduce your chances of eating instead of smoking and the exercise will help to reduce the chance of putting on weight when you stop smoking.
- Keep busy, whether you are at home or at work – the more you've got to do and think about, the less opportunity there is to think about cigarettes.
- If someone offers you a cigarette, tell them very clearly that you're a non-smoker now and ask them not to tempt you again. If they are good friends, they should respect your wish. If they tease you about it, tell you you'll never keep it up and keep offering you more cigarettes, maybe you should see less of them until you are over the first few weeks.
- Accept the fact that it will be hard, that there will be side-effects and unwelcome symptoms. These are entirely normal and they will reduce with time.
- If you really want to see the financial benefits, get a jam-jar and every day put into it the money you would have spent on cigarettes.

It will soon fill up and it won't be long before you can afford to go for a weekend break with your spouse or partner.
- Parties, like pubs, can be danger zones. When you drink you might find it harder to keep your determination up. Be aware of this.

What to do when you are tempted
- Think of the benefits of each cigarette not smoked – a longer life, a healthier life, a more pleasant life, cleaner lungs, blood vessels with fewer clots in them.
- If you have a cigarette you will undo minutes or hours or days or weeks that you've spent off the cigarettes.
- Think of the money you'll start spending again.
- Shut your eyes and remember what your heart attack was like – the fear, the pain, the time in hospital. Ask yourself if you want to increase the risk of that happening again.
- Do something. Go for a walk, have a cup of coffee or tea, have a piece of fruit, go to the loo, go and talk to someone.
- Do your relaxation exercises.
- Do some exercises from your exercise programme.
- Get angry. Get angry with yourself – you're the one that's about to let yourself down. Get angry with the tobacco industry for leading you to this position. Get angry with the government for not banning tobacco.
- If you don't give in, congratulate yourself. You've really done well.
- Whatever happens, tell someone else about it – tell them how difficult it was and how you finally gave in, or were able to weather the storm. If they are good friends they will support you, whatever happened, and just talking about it will help and encourage you.

Always remember that giving up smoking, however many attempts you have to make, is the most valuable thing you can do to reduce your risk of another heart attack.

What to do if you need help
For a start, talk the whole matter over with your family. They are in the best position to help you. Get them to read this chapter, so that they know what is involved in each stage of giving up smoking and can intervene to help if you have a crisis.

Go and see your GP or the cardiac clinic and ask them what help is available. They might be able to help you directly with advice and encouragement and follow-up appointments to see how you're getting on. They might run, or know of, anti-smoking groups or clinics – these could give you support and encouragement when you are feeling vulnerable or if you've suffered a setback and have gone back to smoking for a while.

If you are going to a cardiac rehab programme, tell them that you are giving up smoking and ask what help and advice they can give you. You will be seeing them once or twice a week, and they can provide a strong and regular form of support.

If the craving – the addiction – is very strong you might need the back-up help of nicotine chewing gum or 24-hour skin patches. These can work, although they are certainly not 100 per cent successful. – The bottom line is that you must want to give up first. Skin patches are easier to handle than chewing gum – if you really want a cigarette you chew some gum instead, but it takes 10 minutes or so to remove the craving. However, if you have recently had a heart attack, neither of them might be recommended for you. – Discuss the matter with your GP or preferably at the cardiac clinic.

9 Relaxation and stress management

If you have read this book so far, you will understand that smoking, lack of exercise and eating inappropriate food are the main risk factors for coronary heart disease and heart attacks. Yet a huge number of people who have had heart attacks rate stress – at work, at home, in the family – as somehow being the key factor in precipitating their heart attack. 'Yeah, I know smoking's never done me any good, but it was the pressure at work that tipped my heart over the edge.' Whether you feel this way or not, this chapter is for you. It tells you about stress and about relaxation.

Relaxation and stress are two sides of the same coin. If you feel you suffer from stress, learn how to relax (and it can be easily learned) and you can flip the coin over. In this chapter we will learn about relaxation and some easy ways to become relaxed.

We will also learn about stress – what it is, what it does to you and what you can do to manage it. Relaxation is not always an appropriate strategy if you are at work and feel yourself getting into a stressful situation. Stress management is more about avoiding stressful situations and approaching situations so that they do not appear to be stressful.

Relaxation

Relaxation is crucial to your recovery from a heart attack. The whole process of having a heart attack, being roared into hospital, going into the CCU, then being moved on to the cardiology ward, then being sent home, just as you were getting used to being in hospital, is frightening and stressful. You need to be able to relax, to allow yourself to calm down, to let your body start healing itself, without the distractions of thoughts such as 'What if… ?' 'When will I… ?' 'How can I… ?' All these questions will sort themselves out; you can ask the questions when there are people there to answer them. When you have time to yourself, use it wisely and relax.

In hospital
When you first find yourself in hospital, on the CCU, you will find it

difficult to read – your attention span will be upset, both by what has happened and the drugs that have been run into you. You might find that your vision isn't up to concentrating on books and magazines for a day or so. The best thing your family can do for you is beg, borrow, steal or buy you a Walkman – a personal stereo. Personal CD players are usually not allowed in hospitals – they interfere with the electronic equipment. A personal stereo tape player is what you want, preferably with a built-in FM radio and some good headphones.

Once you've got your Walkman, you're away – if it's got a radio you can listen to whatever station you like – music or talk – and switch off from what's going on around you. If it will only play tapes, get your family to bring in your favourite tapes, get them to borrow tapes off friends and don't forget the taped readings of books.

Ideally, though, you should try to get hold of one or two specific relaxation tapes. Some high street record shops stock them, but a better bet might be a 'New Age' type of shop – it may be the sort of shop that your family or friends might not have been in before, but the staff should know their way around the relaxation tapes available. What you need is not so much a dreamy misty music tape as a guided relaxation tape – for many people relaxation has to be learned and a guided relaxation tape can help enormously. If your local authority runs yoga classes, try and get hold of the telephone number of the yoga teacher; relaxation is an integral part of yoga and the teacher may well be able to give you guidance on what sort of tape to go for.

Once you have got a relaxation tape, use it – maybe a couple of times a day, whether you are in the CCU or on the general cardiology ward. Learning relaxation techniques while you are still in hospital has been shown to improve the recovery process to a significant degree.

At home
When you get home you are going to be off work for some weeks. This book has already given you lots of advice on how to get an exercise and activity programme going right from the first day at home. Alongside this exercise and activity, you must set aside some time each day to relax, preferably once during the morning and once during the afternoon. If you have found a relaxation tape that you are happy with, use this to guide your relaxation. *The Heart Manual*, as already mentioned (see page 129) comes complete with a relaxation tape. However, if you have not found anything that helps you relax, try the following:

- Set aside half-an-hour. Ask that no one comes in to disturb you. Unplug the phone or switch on the answerphone. This is your half-hour. It is part of your reovery programme and is very important, very valuable to you.
- Always use the same room. You need to be able to lie flat on your back, so your bed might be the best bet. Another option is the sitting-room floor.
- Draw the curtains and make certain you are warm. Have a rug over you if necessary.
- Take off your shoes and any other restrictive clothes – your tie, for example. Loosen your belt if it's tight.
- Lie down slowly on your back – don't rush anything. Your legs should be out straight, slightly apart, your feet flopping out. Your arms should be straight, slightly away from your sides, with the palms facing upwards if you can manage that comfortably. No part of your body should be crossing over or touching another part.
- Shut your eyes.
- Breathe in slowly, pushing up your tummy at the same time so the breath goes right down to the bottom of your lungs. Open your mouth and sigh the breath out slowly. Repeat this two or three times. Already you'll be feeling relaxed.
- Tense up the muscles in the right foot for a few seconds, then release all the muscles.
- Tense up the muscles in the right calf – the big muscle behind the shin – hold it for a few seconds, then relax it.
- Tense up the muscles in the right thigh, hold it for a few seconds, then relax.
- Carry out the same procedure on the left foot and leg.
- Tense up both buttocks, hold it for a few seconds, then relax.
- Tense up your tummy muscles for a few seconds, hold it, then relax.
- Arch your back slightly to the ceiling, tensing the muscles, hold it for a few seconds, then relax.
- Stretch out the fingers on your right hand, tensing the muscles, hold it, then relax.
- Tense the muscles in your right forearm, between your wrist and elbow, hold it for a few seconds, then relax.
- Tense the muscles in your right upper arm, hold it, then relax.
- Carry out the same procedure on the left hand and arm.
- Tense up your shoulders so they come up to your ears, hold them like that for a few seconds, then relax them down again.

- Lift up your head slightly, hold it, then relax your neck carefully so that your head sinks back down on to the floor.
- Screw up your face so the muscles are tensed up, hold it, then relax.
- Run your mind slowly up and down your body, checking that all your muscles are relaxed. Do not open your eyes.
- Visualise yourself lying there, almost floating now, completely relaxed, breathing gently.
- Now bring to mind some beautiful warm sunny place. Maybe it's somewhere you know, maybe it's completely imaginary. It might be a garden or a wood or a beach. You are very happy there, very relaxed, very comfortable. You have all the time in the world. Walk around. Look at the flowers, at the trees, at the waves. Be aware of the sounds. Of the smells. Of a slight breeze. Touch a flower, run your hands over a tree trunk, ripple your fingers in the water. Feel the sun warming your skin. Feel yourself relaxed, calm, tranquil, peaceful, content, healthy, happy, at peace with the world and with yourself.
- When you feel you have had enough warmth and peace and relaxation, slowly turn and look at all you can see, and say goodbye to this place. You can come back here whenever you want, it will always be there for you.
- Very slowly get back in touch with your body. Gently move your feet. Gently move your hands. Stretch your legs and arms and relax them. Listen to the sounds of the outside world. Slowly open your eyes, and gently sit up.
- You should be very relaxed. Don't do anything sudden. DO NOT leap to your feet. Take it slowly. Sit and think for a while about where you've been.
- It's quite possible you will go to sleep. This is not a problem. Warn your family that you might go to sleep. If this happens ask them not to wake you suddenly, but to do it quietly – rubbing gently under the ear, next to the jaw bone, is a good way to wake someone up gently.

How you tackle this relaxation session is up to you. You can read it a few times and try to memorise it. You can record it on to a tape then play it back to yourself through your Walkman; if you do this, allow yourself plenty of time between each instruction so that you can carry them out. For the visualisation at the end allow about five minutes before bringing yourself back. Or you can get someone you know well to read the instructions to you.

However you learn it, this is a technique that you can go back to throughout your life, whether it's just the relaxation or the visualisation. As you get used to the sensation of being relaxed, it will become something you can switch into at any time, at any place.

What is stress?

Everyone talks about stress, but what exactly is it? Well, for a start it's not absolute – different people react in different ways to stressful situations. Indeed, a stressful situation for one person – the in-laws coming to stay for a weekend, for example – might be a source of great pleasure and enjoyment to another person.

Very simply, though, if we are exposed to stress we produce the hormone called adrenaline. As already described, adrenaline is responsible for what is known as the 'fight and flight' response. The immediate result of this adrenaline rush is to increase the heart rate, shut down the blood vessels in parts of the body that are not needed to fight or run, e.g. in the gut, and to increase the level of fats (fuel for the fighting or fleeing) in the bloodstream. All this is fine if we actually fight or run, but if we don't we can be left in a state of physical over-excitement that may spill over into the next stressful situation.

What it feels like

A life without excitement would be very dull. That's why we go to fairgrounds, go skiing, go parachuting, drive cars fast, ride motorbikes, go bungy-jumping – the adrenaline rush can be very exciting. But living a life full of stress can be very alarming:

- You feel constantly tense.
- You feel frustrated, always in a bad mood, with sudden outbursts of bad temper or anger.
- You are constantly fearful of things you don't like happening.
- You have difficulty concentrating and remembering things.
- You cannot sleep.
- You can't make decisions and find it particularly difficult deciding to do things.
- You lose your sense of humour.
- You lose your desire for lovemaking, and sometimes you might lose your ability to make love.

What it does to your body

The body's reactions to stress – the reactions you are aware of – are many and varied.

- You have a dry mouth.
- You feel tense, wound up, drawn tight like a stretched elastic band.
- You have butterflies in your tummy.
- You may feel breathless.
- You come out in cold sweats.
- You feel faint or distant.
- Your fingers and toes may tingle or feel peculiar.
- You may be aware of a banging or racing heartbeat or pulse – this is particularly the case if you've had a heart attack and are more aware of what your heart is doing.
- You may suffer from headaches, back aches, shoulder aches, neck aches. These are due to the muscles being tensed up.

Stress management

If you are living a life in which stress is a normal part of the day, these feelings may be with you all the time or most of the time. This is not healthy. It can be frightening. It will seriously hamper your recovery programme after a heart attack. You need to learn how to manage the stress, to avoid it, to 'de-stress' the stressful situations, to use relaxation techniques at crucial moments in the day.

The A and B personalities

We can begin by making a gross generalisation. People are divided into those who cope well with stress and those who don't cope well with stress. As we saw in Chapter 3, people who are submerged by stress are called type A and people who cope with stress are labelled type B. You probably don't fall cleanly into either category, but you may recognise more of your characteristics in one column than another.

Type A	Type B
Competitive.	Not competitive.
Always in a rush.	Always seems to go at their own pace.
No patience.	Very patient.
Doesn't listen well, interrupts.	Good listener.

Hurried talker.	Slow and deliberate when talking.
Doesn't talk about own feelings, inner thoughts.	Does talk about feelings, emotions.
Hurried at other things – eating, walking, domestic chores.	Relaxed at other things – takes but gets them done.
Never late; often early.	Relaxed about time-keeping, but always turns up.
Tries to do many things at once.	Finishes one task before starting another.
Always works at 110 per cent.	Works as hard as is necessary, but always seems relaxed.
Always worried about what others might think.	Concerned about doing things to own satisfaction, not worried about others.
Pushy, ambitious.	Relaxed, easy-going.
Few activities or interests.	Many activities and interests.
Few or no close friends.	Many close friends.

Type A and type B characteristics

If you see yourself as a type A personality (and if you want the truth, ask your family what sort of personality they see you as), then you will help your recovery immeasurably if you can change your life so that you have more type B characteristics. This is not impossible and in the rest of the chapter we will give you some ideas about how it can be done.

Don't think that once a type A personality, always a type A personality. Some changes are quite simple, others more fundamental, but all are possible. But if you keep up the type A habits, there is a risk that sooner or later you will slip back into the sort of life that precipitated your heart attack in the first place.

Give yourself more time
Do you give yourself any time? During the course of a normal day, do you give time to:

- Your work?
- Your work colleagues, both at work and outside work?

- Domestic chores?
- Your spouse/partner?
- Your family?
- Your friends?
- Your acquaintances?
- Yourself? Reading? Hobbies? Exercise? Other activities?

Many people, particularly type A personalities, will tick the first couple of items, maybe the third if they've got a bit of time left over, but the rest will get very little time at all.

What do you do? Answer the questions honestly. Do you really spend time with your spouse or family, relaxing with them, not thinking about other things you should be doing? Do you commit any time to them – say that your time with your family is not going to be eaten into by urgent jobs at work? And yourself? Do you allow yourself any time at all? Time that is not eaten into by other commitments?

But what's this got to do with managing stress, you might be asking? Quite a lot, in fact. At its very simplest, taking time off, time out, time relaxing, whatever you want to call it, provides you with a buffer, a period when your body and mind can unwind, when you can step off the treadmill. This treadmill is an important image – many people who suffer from stress feel that they are on a treadmill, that they have no control over it, that they are stuck on it, caged in. But this is not the case. You can take time off.

Set a period of the week – say Saturday afternoon – aside, and agree with yourself and your family that you will accept no commitments during that time. It's your 'playtime' if you like. Then write down a list of everything you'd like to do on the Saturday afternoons – it might be gardening, it might be going to the football, it might be visits to other members of the family, it might be all sorts of things. Make the list as long as you like, throw in some ideas that might seem childish or irresponsible. Put the list on the fridge – use a fridge magnet to stick it there.

Now comes the difficult bit. Don't plan anything to begin with. Get to Saturday, or whatever day you've chosen, and see what seems like a good idea. It's pouring with rain? How about a movie or a trip to see the children? Sunny weather? How about an afternoon in the country or at the zoo with the grandkids or in the garden? Don't know what to do? Don't do anything. Or go to bed. When did you last spend an afternoon in bed with your wife or husband or partner?

The important thing is to set that period aside and take on no other commitments, and to do this you might have to learn to say 'No'. 'No, I'm not going to go into work on a Saturday afternoon.' 'No I'm not going to do that mending now.' 'No, I'm not going to make you a sandwich now.' People might get crabby with you at first – 'But we always do the shopping on Saturday afternoon!' – but once they realise that you're serious, that this is your time off the treadmill, that it's 'playtime', they'll leave you alone and respect your decision. And keep in mind that image of stepping off the treadmill.

Controlling the load

When your GP and you agree that you can go back to work, it means just that – you can go back to a normal day's work. If that normal day is chock-a-block full of work and you enjoy it and don't end up feeling tense and angry and panicky and fed up, then you obviously cope with it very well and it doesn't stress you out. Fine.

But a lot of people have a lot to do and they don't cope well. Everything's always in a rush, a panic, they feel that they're only just holding on to things – there's so much to do, all at once, and it's impossible to tell what to do first. If you are like this, you need to sit down, take some deep relaxing breaths and slowly work out what needs doing when.

- Draw up a list of all the jobs that need doing.
- Prioritise them – decide which is most important and which is least important and number the ones in between in order.
- Give them all deadlines and make them realistic deadlines. When your boss said 'Do it now', what did he mean? In an hour's time? Today? Tomorrow morning?

Now go through the list and see if it's practicable for you to do all the jobs within their deadlines. Yes? Well then, tackle them in order of deadline and/or importance, and try not to start one until the previous one is finished. But if you don't stand a hope in hell of doing all the jobs within the expected deadlines, then you need to take some action:

- Are there any jobs that can go, that you can ignore? If so, ignore them.
- Are there any jobs that someone else should be doing? If so, hand

them back, firmly and politely, and say that you can't do them after all.

- If you still feel that there is too much to do in the time set, ask to see your boss and discuss the matter with them. A solution may not pop up immediately, but a problem shared is a problem halved.

People who are self-employed are in the hardest position from this point of view, because they are their own bosses. There is the fear that this job might be the last, that the work will dry up, that the money will run out. They have to look at their workload and be even more ruthless about sorting out deadlines and priorities than an employee, and once a decision is made it has to be stuck to. 'Oh, but where will the money come from if I don't take on all this work?' The question perhaps ought to be 'Where will the money come from if I kill myself from overwork?'

Some people manage to get through an incredible amount each day going flat-out:

- They rush through their meals or eat them on the run or completely miss them.
- They drive everywhere at 90 miles an hour.
- No sooner have they finished one job than they start another one.
- They cut corners in their work, always concerned about doing things quickly and not necessarily concerned about doing things well.

If you can work like this, do a good job that you and your colleagues are satisfied with, and remain relaxed and happy, fine. But most people who work like this are working on the edge – if one thing goes wrong they lose their temper, get angry, complain about being burdened with idiots. They are working at the limit of their stress threshold.

If you feel you work like this, there are various strategies you can employ. For a start, go back and draw up your list of jobs, deadlines and priorities. Look at the deadlines. Add 10 per cent to each of them if you can. When you make an appointment to see someone, allow more time for the journey. Is the previous appointment likely to over-run? Allow for this as well. When you finish a job, take a break, maybe just for a cup of tea; give yourself enough time to assess whether you've done a good job and not rushed it. This may sound anarchic, but allow yourself to daydream for a few minutes during the day or spend a few minutes every now and then relaxing – it'll recharge your reserves and won't remove a huge chunk from your productive day.

You may describe yourself as hard-working. But look closely at what you're doing. Is it hard work or does it go over the top? Hard work will not kill you and it certainly won't increase your risk of a heart attack. But going over the top is something else. That is when you have no other interests apart from your work, or if you do they become obsessive as well; some people who go over the top at work take up an activity like squash or golf, then go over the top with that as well, devoting all their spare time to getting to the top of the local league table or constantly to reducing their handicap. Do you work yourself into the ground, choosing to stay on at the office until well into the evening, choosing to work rather than see the grandchildren in their Christmas play, taking on two part-time jobs as well as doing all the housework? Are you going over the top?

The chances are you'll answer, 'No'. Being a workaholic is like being an alcoholic; neither admit to their problem.

To stop yourself going over the top you have to make some pretty fundamental changes. For a start, you have to realise that your body is not designed to be run flat-out, always teetering on the edge of an adrenaline overdose. It has to have its periods of rest and relaxation, otherwise it gets increasingly sick – your heart attack might have been a sign of this problem. You have to allow more time into your life – time for yourself, for your family, for your friends, for your rest and relaxation. You might have to be less ambitious; what price have you had to pay for ambitions achieved? Ask yourself, have you ever been truly satisfied with the ambitions you've achieved? Was the price worth it? Is it worth chasing yet more personal ambitions – more money, a bigger car, a bigger house – if you're always working so hard you never get a chance to enjoy them.

Having a heart attack gives you a view of your mortality. It might be frightening for you. It will certainly provoke you into thinking about your life and its priorities. Look upon it as a heaven-sent opportunity to reduce the stress levels in your life. If you suddenly announced that you weren't prepared to work until eight every evening, your colleagues might take exception to your unilateral decision. Or maybe you decide that you're not going to do all the cooking and washing up and hoovering on your own. But if you use your heart attack as a cue to discuss the working hours or the domestic chores, then people are likely to be more sympathetic (particularly if you point out that it might be them next time). This is not suggesting that you hide behind the fact of your heart attack – you use it as a cue. 'Listen, since my heart attack I've had a chance to think about what I'm doing, and I'm not happy with it. I don't want to give up my work, but I want some more time with my family/I want more time to myself/I don't want to work at these stress levels. What do you lot think?'

As was pointed out at the beginning of this book, if you want to avoid another heart attack, you need to make some fundamental changes to your life and these changes need to stick with you for the rest of your life. These changes don't just apply to food and exercise and smoking. They apply to your whole life. It does not mean you have to give up working (although if that's what you want, see if you can manage it without crippling yourself financially), but it may well mean that you will have to look at the way you approach work and play, and change some of your priorities. This is not hard, once you've made the decision to do it. This chapter has given you some tools with which to achieve this change.

10 Food and weight

Note that this chapter is not called 'Diet', or 'Dieting', or 'Low-Fat Diet' – in fact the word 'diet' hardly crops up in the chapter at all. This is a chapter on *food* – on what you should be eating if you want to reduce your risk of another heart attack and if you need to reduce your weight. If you have a serious blood cholesterol problem and you are advised to go on a cholesterol-lowering diet, then that is a different matter and there are specific books that can help (Vermilion publish *Cholesterol – Lowering Your Risk*, by David Symes and the FHA, and *The FHA Low-Fat Diet Book* by David Symes, Annette Zakary and Angela Dickinson).

The very simplest advice on food that can be offered can be summarised in eight positive points.

1   Do enjoy your food.
2   Do make certain you get enough vitamins and minerals by eating plenty of fruit and vegetables.
3   Do eat plenty of foods that are high in starch and fibre – bread, potatoes, pasta, rice.
4   Do eat the right amount to be a healthy weight.
5   Do cut down on the fatty foods.
6   Do cut down on the sugary foods.
7   Do eat a variety of different foods – not chips with everything every day.
8   If you drink, do keep within sensible limits, whether it's tea, coffee or alcohol.

If you remember nothing else from this chapter, remember and act on these eight points.

Cholesterol

If you have had a heart attack then various features of your health will be monitored for the rest of your life. Your blood cholesterol level is one of these features. We have looked at the role of cholesterol as a risk factor in coronary heart disease in Chapter 3; here we will summarise some of those details.

Cholesterol is a fat that is found in all the cells of the body. It is essential to life. It is transported around the body in the bloodstream and it is when the levels of cholesterol in the bloodstream get too high that we have problems. High levels of blood cholesterol contribute significantly to the furring up of arteries and thus to coronary heart disease and to the risk of a heart attack; for every 1 per cent that the blood cholesterol level is raised, there is a 2 per cent increase in the risk of coronary heart disease.

The blood cholesterol level is directly linked with the amount of fat we consume, particularly with the amount of saturated fat. The amount of dietary cholesterol we consume is largely irrelevant. As a gross generalisation, we all eat too much fat, we all eat too much saturated fat and as a result, as a population, we all have high blood cholesterol levels.

But what is the generally recommended level? Blood cholesterol levels are measured in units called millimoles per litre, abbreviated to mmol/l: In general:

- Below 5.2 mmol/l is the ideal. If you have other risk factors such as smoking, being overweight or having high blood pressure, you should be advised by your GP to do something about them, but in general if you have a cholesterol level below 5.2 you will be sent on your way with a smile.
- Between 5.2 and 6.4 mmol/l is seen as a mild problem. You should be advised on healthy eating and exercise, as well as on any other risk factors you may have. You should heed this advice.
- Between 6.5 and 7.8 mmol/l is seen as a more serious problem, and advice on diet, exercise and other risk factors for coronary heart disease should be more emphatic and detailed. Underlying causes of the problem should be sought by your doctor and addressed.
- Over 7.8 mmol/l is a severe problem and should be addressed with specialist advice, perhaps involving a dietitian and appointments at a lipid clinic.

Your blood cholesterol level is usually assessed by testing a small sample of blood that is withdrawn from a vein in your arm. There are now a range of machines available that can give you a reading in a matter of minutes, using a pinprick blood sample. It is now even possible to measure your cholesterol level using a home testing kit. Such readings should always be followed up with advice from a doctor and subsequent testing to confirm or add more detail to the initial result. If you have such a test, the advice is always to go and see your GP if you are in any way concerned or unsure about what it means.

The next section of this chapter looks at how you can help keep your blood cholesterol level within healthy limits.

The four food groups

There are many books and leaflets on the market that give detailed advice on what to eat and what not to eat if you want to bring your cholesterol level down and reduce your risk of coronary heart disease. What is suggested here is a simple method of dividing up the various foods you eat and eating more of some than of others. Unless you have a serious cholesterol or weight problem, the advice is not to give anything up, merely to eat more of some foods than others.

So, what are these food groups and what amounts should we eat each day?

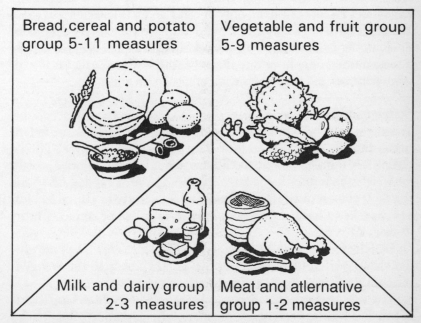

Bread, cereal and potato group 5-11 measures

Vegetable and fruit group 5-9 measures

Milk and dairy group 2-3 measures

Meat and atlernative group 1-2 measures

Fig. 10 *The four food groups.*

- Starchy foods – bread, cereals and potatoes. We should eat 5 to 11 portions each day.
- Vegetables and fruit – fresh, frozen, tinned or preserved. We should eat 5 to 9 portions each day.
- Lean meat, poultry, fish. We should eat 1 to 2 portions each day.
- Low-fat dairy produce – milk, butter/spreads, cheese, yoghurt. We should eat 2 to 3 portions each day.

There is a summary table later in this chapter that gives slightly more detail about what foods are involved in the different groups and what a portion is in each case. But what should be obvious is that the emphasis should be on eating more starchy foods – bread, potatoes, pasta, rice, dried lentils, dried beans – and more fruit and vegetables, and less meat, poultry, fish, milk, cheese and other dairy produce.

Again, the point has to be made that you don't have to give up some foods completely, merely cut back on some and eat more of others. If you fry food, get a non-stick frying pan and use a small quantity (a teaspoon is usually enough) of appropriate oil – monounsaturated or polyunsaturated. If you like bacon and eggs for breakfast, fine, but it is sensible to have them less frequently, say only at weekends, and perhaps have fewer rashers of bacon, only one egg and a thicker slice of toast. You don't have to give up chips, but don't have them every day; go for the lower-fat oven varieties if you cook them at home. When you have a roast dinner, only have one slice of meat, and make up for it with more potatoes and vegetables and perhaps extra gravy.

Starch and fibre
You might have been brought up to think that starchy foods are fattening – they're stodgy, therefore they must make you fat. This is completely untrue. Starchy foods have about half the calories, weight for weight, that fatty foods have, providing you don't add fat to the starch. If you eat more starchy foods and fewer fatty foods you feel just as full, take in fewer calories and lower your risk of coronary heart disease, all in one go.

Starchy foods are also a very good source of energy. They are ultimately converted to glucose, but this occurs slowly so the energy is released slowly to keep us going throughout the day.

The starchy foods are a very good source of fibre. Fibre has all sorts of benefits: it helps prevent constipation; it helps prevent piles; it helps prevent other digestive disorders, including cancer of the gut; it helps prevent diabetes; and it helps prevent coronary heart disease.

Most starchy foods are cheap, easy to prepare and can help to stretch main meals and small amounts of expensive ingredients.

About half of each meal should consist of starchy foods, whether it's cereals and toast at breakfast, bread for sandwiches at lunchtime, or potatoes, pasta or rice for the evening meal.

So, what are the starchy foods? Well, they are many and varied.

- Bread is the obvious one. Everyone eats bread. Everyone should eat more bread. Eat different types of bread – wholemeal, granary, white, oat loaf, mixed grain. There are so many varieties. Experiment and discover how tasty some of them are. Cut the slices thick and use less spread. Go for the low-fat spreads, or use cottage cheese or chutneys to moisten your lunchtime sandwiches. (If you're used to buying sliced bread, you might have to invest in a bread knife, although many bakeries and supermarkets will slice loaves for you if you ask. Ask them to slice the loaf into thick slices.)
- Then there are potatoes. You can cook potatoes in many ways – boiled, mashed, jacket, roast, fried, chips. Get used to eating them with less fat on them. Put low-fat yoghurt or fromage frais or lemon juice or Worcester sauce on jacket potatoes, not butter. Put gravy on boiled potatoes instead of butter; mash potatoes with more milk and less fat, and use polyunsaturated or monounsaturated margarine instead of butter, fry potatoes in less oil; buy low-fat oven chips; roast potatoes in less oil.
- Pasta is featuring more and more on the menu at home. There are all sorts of different varieties – spaghetti, tubes, twists, shells, bow-tie shapes, coloured pasta, wholemeal pasta, fresh pasta, dried pasta. Go more for the tomato-based sauces, not so much the creamy or oily sauces. Cook pasta in baked dishes, with fish for example. Sprinkle a bit of Parmesan cheese on top – it gives a good flavour without too much fat.
- Rice can accompany many meals, not just curries. It works with stews and casseroles, as well as fricassees, goulashes and hotpots. And don't forget rice puddings.
- Other cereals are available in the supermarkets now – cous-cous and bulgar wheat, for example. They are easy to cook and can be used instead of rice and pasta in many meals.
- Lentils, dried split peas, dried beans, e.g. red beans, are all starchy

foods, with the addition of protein, and can all be bought in the supermarkets. They are either easily cooked or can be found ready cooked in tins. Use them to extend meals cheaply, thus adding extra starch and fibre.

- Breakfast cereals are a good form of starch and fibre. Go for the higher fibre varieties, and try to avoid the sugar-coated ones. Do not smother them with sugar – add chopped fresh fruit, stewed fruit or dried fruit to sweeten them instead. Eat them with semi-skimmed milk or with low-fat yoghurt or fromage frais.
- When did you last have porridge for breakfast? This is a delicious low-fat/high-fibre meal. Make it with skimmed or semi-skimmed milk for a creamier flavour. Mix in raisins or sultanas to provide a sweeter taste.

Fruit and vegetables

Fruit and vegetables should be an important part of everyone's food, but unfortunately for the nation's health people eat far too few. Many people could double their intake of fruit and vegetables, and still only just eat enough.

Fruit and vegetables are one of the most important sources of vitamins and minerals – those essential ingredients that help keep us healthy. Not only do vitamins and minerals keep some specific diseases at bay, but they are important for our ability to combat all infections and diseases.

Fruit and vegetables are another good source of dietary fibre, and we have seen in the previous section on starchy foods how important dietary fibre is.

If you are trying to lose weight or not eat so much, fruit and vegetables are very important. They can fill you up, but have even fewer calories than starchy foods. Celery is famous in this respect; you use up more calories chewing it and digesting it than it provides. Here are some guidelines on fruit and vegetables:

- You can eat as much of them as you like, even if you are trying to lose weight.
- You should aim to eat some fruit or vegetable, cooked or raw, with every meal, even breakfast. If you normally have no breakfast, try a piece of fruit – an apple or a banana.
- Eat as wide a variety of fruit and vegetables as you can, to get the full range of vitamins and minerals.

- Don't just think of fresh fruit and vegetables – frozen and tinned varieties can be just as good, although go for the tinned vegetables that are low in salt and the tinned fruit that is in water or natural juice, not syrup.
- Vegetables don't need gallons of water to cook them in, just a little. Or try steaming them or cooking them in the microwave.
- Stir fry sliced vegetables in a little oil. Sliced fish or meat can then be added to make a full meal.
- A very wide range of salads can be dreamed up or look at the hundreds of salad recipes that are in cookery books and magazines. Dress them with just a little oil, with lemon juice or vinegar, or with a low-fat yoghurt or fromage frais.
- If you are used to snacking during the day – at elevenses, or at an afternoon tea break – eat some fruit instead of a packet of crisps or a chocolate bar. The fruit is often cheaper, has far fewer calories, is just as tasty and does you more good.

Fat

There is probably more confusion over fat than over any other aspect of our food. The basic advice, though, couldn't be simpler: eat less fat. But what a lot of people don't realise is quite how much fat is in our food already. All the following items have a high fat content:

- Fatty cuts of meat.
- Animal skin, e.g. bacon rind, chicken skin.
- Most processed meats, e.g. sausages, pâtés, salamis, luncheon meats.
- Cream and full-fat (silver or gold top) milk.
- Butter and margarine – even most of the low-fat spreads have a high fat content, although less than, say, butter.
- Suet, lard and dripping.
- Full-fat yoghurt and fromage frais.
- Most cheeses.
- Pastries, biscuits, cakes, puddings, chocolate bars and other sweet snacks.
- Crisps and other savoury snacks.
- Fried foods.

Remember, the advice is to eat *less* fat. So it's not a question of giving up these foods, merely of eating less of them and then switching to low-fat or lower-fat alternatives made with mono-unsaturates and/or polyunsaturates. But what are these different types of fat?

- Saturated fats (saturates) and trans-fatty acids are the bad fats. They give rise to raised blood cholesterol levels and increase the risk of your arteries furring up. Saturated fats are largely of animal origin (and this includes the fats found in dairy produce), while trans-fatty acids are a product of food processing.
- Polyunsaturated fats (polyunsaturates) are largely of vegetable origin and do not give rise to raised cholesterol levels. Many food products are now available made with polyunsaturates.
- Mono-unsaturated fats (mono-unsaturates) are also largely of vegetable origin. They do not give rise to raised cholesterol levels. But what they can do in some situations is to raise the level of 'good' HDL cholesterol in the blood. Because of this, mono-unsaturates are now seen as giving you some protection against coronary heart disease. This does not mean you should gobble down as many mono-unsaturated fats as possible. The advice is still to reduce the fat intake – but where possible to use mono-unsaturates.

Mono-unsaturates	Polyunsaturates	Saturates and trans-fatty acids
Olive oil	Sunflower oil	Palm oil
Peanut (groundnut) oil	Safflower oil	Coconut oil
Rapeseed oil	Corn oil	Butter
Margarines and spreads labelled high in mono-unsaturates	Soya oil	Lard
	Walnut oil	Hard margarine
	Margarines and spreads labelled high in polyunsaturates	Suet
		Vegetarian suet
		Standard soft margarine

Classification of cooking oils and fats

All fats contain a mixture of these three groups – saturates (and trans-fatty acids), polyunsaturates and mono-unsaturates. Furthermore, all processed foods now have to be labelled with a breakdown of fats, carbohydrates, proteins and other food groups. You should aim to buy products that are labelled low in saturates (and trans-fatty acids) and high in polyunsaturates and mono-unsaturates.

So, to summarise the advice on fats:

- Reduce the fat intake – this is the most important piece of advice.
- Saturates should comprise the smallest proportion of fats – this is the next most important piece of advice.
- Where possible, buy foodstuffs that are labelled high in mono-unsaturates.
- Where possible, buy foodstuffs that are labelled high in polyunsaturates.
- When cooking use small amounts of mono-unsaturated or polyunsaturated oil when necessary.

The following tips will help you reduce your fat intake without your having to change your eating habits drastically:

- Grill, steam, poach or casserole your food rather than frying it.
- Go for the leaner cuts of meat.
- Trim the excess fat off meat whenever you can.
- Go for lean mince, now widely available.
- Eat more fish, twice a week if you can – fish, particularly oily fish, gives you good protection against the arteries furring up.
- Eat more chicken, but remove the skin whenever you can.
- Use skimmed milk for cooking, for tea and coffee, and semi-skimmed milk for cereals.
- Use low-fat spreads instead of butter and try to get varieties that are labelled high in mono-unsaturates or high in polyunsaturates.
- Try different low-fat spreads until you find one that you like.
- Cut bread in thicker slices and spread the low-fat spread thinly – more bread, less spread.
- Some low-fat spreads look dreadful on hot toast, because of their high water content. If this is the case, simply let the toast cool before using the spread.
- Try using low-fat spread on only one slice of a sandwich and perhaps put chutney on the other slice. If it's a particularly moist and tasty sandwich filling, try doing without the low-fat spread completely.
- When you do fry food, use the bare minimum of a mono-

unsaturated or polyunsaturated oil (a teaspoon is usually enough).

- Get cooking oil that is labelled high in mono-unsaturates (rape-seed oil is the cheapest) or high in polyunsaturates (sunflower or safflower oil).
- Go for low-fat cheese (cottage cheese) or reduced-fat cheese instead of ordinary cheese.
- If you need a strong cheesey flavour in a recipe, use a small quantity of a high-fat strongly flavoured cheese, like a mature cheddar or Parmesan.
- When eggs are used in recipes, try using two egg whites for one egg, and give the yolk to your cat or dog (the egg yolk contains all the fat in eggs, the egg white contains none).
- Try and reduce the number of meals based on meat pies, sausages, burgers, salamis, smoked sausages and luncheon meats, as they are all high in fat – usually saturated fat.
- Have fruit or a low-fat yoghurt or fromage frais for snacks instead of crisps, savoury snacks, chocolate bars, biscuits, cake, etc.
- Have slices of malt loaf, a fruit scone or a currant bun, all unbuttered, instead of biscuits or cake.
- In salad dressing, cut down the amount of oil and increase the amount of lemon juice or vinegar. Add a bit of French mustard to give a bit more flavour.
- Instead of full-fat salad cream or mayonnaise, use low-fat varieties, or use low-fat yoghurt or fromage frais with some lemon juice stirred into it.
- For chips, get low-fat oven chips.
- For roast potatoes use the bare minimum of oil and go for an oil that is high in mono-unsaturates or polyunsaturates.
- Go for jacket potatoes or mashed potatoes, or rice or pasta, instead of chips or roast potatoes.
- On your jacket potatoes, don't use butter or margarine; instead try low-fat yoghurt or fromage frais, or tomato ketchup, or Worcestershire sauce, or barbecue sauce – the possibilities are endless.
- Make mashed potatoes with more skimmed milk and less butter or margarine, or try using low-fat yoghurt or fromage frais instead.
- Try using low-fat yoghurt or fromage frais on your puddings instead of cream or custard.
- Try making sauces with cornflour instead of butter/margarine and flour.

It cannot be emphasised enough that the idea is not to switch to a completely new diet, but to modify your foods and cooking to reduce your intake of fat, in particular your intake of saturated fats.

Sugar

Sugar does not play a direct role in the risk of coronary heart disease. However, most people consume a lot of sugar, either directly on cereals, and in tea and coffee, or indirectly in biscuits, cakes, cooked puddings and processed foods and snacks. This increases the chance of being overweight and being overweight is a risk factor for coronary heart disease.

In fact, we don't need to eat sugar at all – it's a myth. We can get all the energy we need from the starchy foods and the fat we eat. And eating sugary foods is certainly the main cause of tooth decay.

It therefore makes sense to try and reduce your consumption of sugar.

- Brown sugar, Demerara sugar, syrup, honey, maple syrup are just the same as sugar and are no 'healthier'.
- Try to give up taking sugar in tea and coffee or use one of the artificial sweeteners.
- Drink mineral water or low-calorie fizzy drinks instead of squash or ordinary fizzy drinks.
- Cut down on cakes, biscuits, chocolate bars and sweet snacks bars – not only are they high in sugar, but they're usually high in fat as well, so you'll be doing yourself a double favour. Instead, eat fruit for snacks, or an unbuttered currant bun or fruit scone or slice of malt loaf, or a low-fat yoghurt.
- If you do buy biscuits, try and get those that are lower in sugar and fat.
- Choose breakfast cereals that are not coated with sugar or loaded with chocolate. Get the non-sweetened ones and try them with slices of fresh fruit or dried fruit instead of sprinkling sugar over them.
- Go for the reduced sugar jams and marmalades, or use other spreads like Marmite or cottage cheese that are low in sugar and fat.
- If you buy tinned fruit, get the ones in water or fruit juice, not in syrup.
- Many savoury foods have high sugar contents, e.g. pickles, chutneys, ketchup and sauces. Get low-sugar varieties if they are available or simply use them in small quantities.

Salt

The intake of sodium has a direct impact on blood pressure and high blood pressure is a risk factor for coronary heart disease. The major input of sodium in our food is from ordinary salt – sodium chloride. It therefore makes sense to try and limit the amount of salt we eat, particularly if you have already had a heart attack. If you also have high blood pressure, this advice is very, very important.

The recommended intake of salt per person each day is about 6 grams (0.2 oz). The average person in the UK in fact consumes about 10 grams (0.3 oz) of salt a day, over a third of an ounce, and the majority of this comes from processed and convenience food – the ready prepared food and meals bought in the shops. Cutting down on salt added at the table or in the kitchen is one way of reducing the salt intake; careful shopping is equally important, though. However, it has to be accepted that salt in food is a habit and it is difficult to break this habit overnight. Aim to cut down gradually. Here are some tips.

- Always taste food before adding salt. Don't add salt as a matter of routine.
- On food labels salt will be listed as 'sodium chloride' and as 'monosodium glutamate'. Try and avoid foods that have a high concentration of either of these.
- Canned/packet soups, savoury snacks, 'pot' noodles and bought sauces all tend to be high in salt. Try to prepare home-cooked alternatives when possible – they'll probably be cheaper as well as healthier.
- Go for fresh fruit and vegetables – tomatoes, celery, carrots, broccoli pieces – instead of salty snacks such as crisps and other savouries.
- Go for unsalted nuts and raisins rather than salted or dry roast nuts.
- Limit your consumption of salted meats like bacon, ham and salami.
- Use less salt in your cooking and at the table. Add extra flavour by using herbs, spices or lemon juice.
- If you really miss the taste of salt, try the low-salt alternatives, but note that low-salt alternatives should not be used if you suffer from any kidney condition.

Drinks

The simple advice is drink plenty of fluids – 3 litres (5 pints) a day, about 10 mugs, is what is recommended. Some of this fluid will be consumed as part of your food, e.g. milk on cereals, but most people in this country drink far less than this amount. You don't have to go out of your way to make endless cups of tea – in fact this will probably do more harm than good. Drink water instead. The water from the taps is safe and cheap, while bottled water is just as safe, if a little more expensive. Here are some other tips:

- Caffeine is found in tea, coffee and cola drinks. In large quantities it can make you feel restless and anxious, and can result in sleeplessness. It makes sense to limit your consumption of these drinks or choose caffeine-free varieties, especially towards the end of the day.
- Many drinks contain high levels of sugar. You might think that three spoonsful of sugar in tea or coffee is a lot, but many fizzy drinks have five or six spoonsful of sugar in them. Neither sugar in tea/coffee nor sugar in fizzy drinks does your weight any good and it will encourage tooth decay. Try and avoid sugar if you can or choose non-sugar sweeteners.
- Go for pure fruit juices, although not in large quantities. They have no added sugar and are based on fruit juice concentrates, so they are rich in fruit sugar (fructose). Fruit drinks (often in boxes looking very like fruit juice boxes) invariably have added sugar.
- Alcoholic drinks tend to be very high in calories, and too much alcohol can do your health no good. The recommended levels are up to 21 units per week for men and up to 14 units per week for women, a unit being a half-pint (a quarter of a litre) of beer, a single shot of spirits or a small glass of wine.

Eating meals
There is a tremendous temptation when adjusting your food, particularly if you are trying to lose weight or are busy, to eat small or non-existent breakfasts and lunches, then to have a large meal at the end of the day. For all sorts of reasons, the advice is to eat three proper meals a day:

- Eat a proper two-course breakfast, sitting down. Don't rush through the meal.
- Eat a proper lunch, again sitting down. It might be a sandwich lunch or a meal on a plate – at home or in the works canteen – but make certain it's a two-course meal. Again, don't rush it.
- The evening meal might be smaller because you've eaten breakfast and lunch, but again ensure it is a two-course sit-down meal.

A two-course meal might sound like an extravagance for breakfast or lunch, but it needn't be such a big deal: a bowl of cereal and fruit, followed by some toast, for breakfast; maybe a couple of rounds of sandwiches followed by a piece of fruit for lunch. There are many advantages to having three proper meals like this each day, some of them obvious, some less obvious:

- If you eat three meals a day you will digest your food better. Eating very little during the day, then a large meal in the evening, overloads the digestive system at just the time it should be slowing down for the night.
- Eating three meals a day means you will have less need or desire for snacks during the day. As bought snacks tend to be high in fat and sugar, this will tend to reduce your fat and sugar intake.
- If you are snacking less and eating three main meals that you or your partner or spouse have control over, you give yourself more opportunity to implement advice on sensible eating.
- Having sit-down meals can give you some time to yourself or with your family or friends.
- Having sit-down meals can allow you to unwind, to reduce your stress level, to relax.

Summary
The table opposite summarises the main points of this section.

Eating out

Eating out is a pleasure most of us enjoy. It might be a stop at a fast-food outlet or it might be an occasion to celebrate at a restaurant. On average, in the UK we eat out twice a week. And when we do, what we want is food that is both tasty and sensible. To meet these two requirements does not mean that you have to forego the enjoyment and socialising involved in eating out; good choices are available in most places, though you have to be aware of what exactly it is you are ordering, and if necessary ask questions and make requests.

If you are calling the restaurant in advance to make a reservation, you can check whether they can cater for special requests. At the restaurant do not be intimidated by the menu or the staff. Ask questions about the ingredients of dishes and the way they are cooked, and request alterations in either of them, if need be – the cook will usually

Food group	Daily portions	What is a portion?
Bread, cereal, potato group	5 to 11 Eat some wholegrain products daily.	3 tbsp breakfast cereal, or 1 slice toast/bread, or $\frac{1}{2}$ a bread roll/bun, or 3 to 4 cracker biscuits, or 2 tbsp cooked rice/pasta/noodles, or 1 egg-sized potato.
Vegetable, fruit group	5 to 9 Include a variety of fruit and vegetables daily.	2 tbsp vegetables, or 1 small portion of salad, or 1 piece of fresh fruit, or 2 tbsp cooked/tinned fruit, or 100-ml (small box) fruit juice.
Milk, dairy group	2 to 3 Choose low/ lower-fat varieties.	$\frac{1}{2}$ pint milk, or 1 small pot of yoghurt/fromage frais, or 1 oz/25 grams cheese (size of a small matchbox).
Meat, alternatives group	1 to 2	2–3 oz/60–90 grams lean meat/ poultry without skin/oily fish, or 4–5 oz/100–130 grams white fish (not fried), or 2 eggs (up to 3–4 each week), or 6 oz/200 grams cooked beans/ chickpeas/lentils, or 2 tbsp/2 oz/60 grams nuts
Fats	3 maximum	1 tsp butter, or 2 tsp low-fat spread, or 1 tsp oil (mono- or polyunsaturated), or 1 tsp mayonnaise/oily salad dressing
Fatty foods, cakes, sweets	1 maximum	Fatty meat or sausages or luncheon meat or crisps or biscuits or rich sauces or fatty gravies or cream or cream cheese or pastries or pies or cakes or doughnuts or rich/dairy ice cream.

Summary of healthy food choices

173

be perfectly happy to please. Ask for sauces or dressings on the side, so that you can choose how much you take. If you want to cut down the portion size, choose a starter as a main course or ask for an extra plate and share a main course with one of your companions.

When studying a menu, the following terms usually mean a healthier option:

- Baked – cooked in a dry heat, in the oven.
- Braised – pot-cooked food in its own juices.
- Broiled – similar to grilled.
- Casseroled.
- Char-grilled – grilled to blacken or to scorch the surface of the food.
- Dry broiled.
- Flame cooked.
- Garden fresh.
- Grilled.
- In its own juice.
- Lightly tossed (usually a salad).
- Marinated.
- Microwaved – this usually means that no fat is used.
- Poached.
- Steamed.
- Stewed.
- Stir-fried.

In contrast, the following terms often mean extra fat (and therefore extra calories):

- A la crème – with cream, creamy.
- Alfredo – as the cook chooses.
- Au gratin – with cheese, cheesy.
- Batter dipped, battered.
- Béarnaise – in a rich sauce made with egg yolks, butter and other ingredients.
- Béchamel – a thick white sauce flavoured with onion and seasoning.
- Beurre blanc – white sauce with butter as an ingredient.
- Breaded – may be fried after it is breaded.
- Buttery, buttered, in butter sauce.
- Cheese sauce.

- Cordon bleu – food prepared to a high standard, which could be very rich.
- Creamed, in a cream sauce, in its own gravy.
- Crispy – usually means fried.
- Deep fried.
- En croûte – in pastry.
- Escalloped – covered in egg and then breadcrumbed, then fried; may be served with a rich sauce.
- Flaky.
- Florentine eggs.
- Fried.
- Hollandaise – a rich sauce made with egg yolks, butter and other ingredients.
- Meunière – dredged with flour, then fried in butter.
- Milanese – butter likely to be an ingredient.
- Pan fried.
- Parmigiona – Parmesan cheese or Parma ham/proscuitto likey to be used.
- Puffed.
- Rich.
- Sauté – fried.
- Smothered in.
- Tempura – dipped in batter and deep fried.

Weight

We have already looked at weight as a risk factor for coronary heart disease and heart attacks in Chapter 3. This section overlaps with that earlier material.

Are you overweight?
Being overweight is being over a defined ideal weight for your height and sex, and various studies have demonstrated that there is a direct increase in one's risk of coronary heart disease with increase in weight above one's ideal weight. If you have already had a heart attack, then you have probably discussed what is your ideal weight with your GP, with the staff at the cardiac clinic or with the cardiac rehab staff. If this hasn't occurred, it would be wise to bring the matter up. It might be that there is no problem, you are well within the limits for your ideal weight, and that's the end of the matter. If a problem is identified

with your weight it will then be possible to work out a strategy together for getting your weight down.

But how do you begin to work out whether you are overweight or not? There are all sorts of methods and tables and charts that can be used to determine this.

- The simplest merely correlate weight with height and state that if you are a man or woman of such-and-such a height, then you ought to weigh so much.

- A more realistic assessment is to accept that there are bound to be variations in the population and to provide a chart that tells you for a given height what range of weight might indicate whether you are underweight, satisfactory, overweight or obese.

- There is a the body – mass index, or BMI (also known as the Quetelet index). This is recommended by many authorities as being the best indicator. In practice, the BMI can most conveniently be measured from a chart, which also usually indicates the relative risk of coronary heart disease associated with different levels of being overweight:

  A BMI of 20 or less indicates being underweight.
  A BMI of 20–25 indicates an acceptable level.
  A BMI of 25–30 indicates being overweight, i.e. some health risk.
  A BMI of 30–40 indicates obesity, i.e. moderate health risk.
  A BMI of over 40 indicates severe obesity, i.e. high health risk.

- There is the waist-to-hip ratio, i.e. waist measurement divided by the hip measurement. A high waist:hip ratio indicates an increased risk of coronary heart disease; for women 'high' is over 0.8, while for men it is over 1.

- A completely different assessment is to measure the thickness of a fold of skin. Above a certain thickness in a specific part of the body indicates that deposits of fat exist under the skin. As one loses weight, so this skin-fold will get thinner.

Statistics show that about 45 per cent of the UK population is overweight, and 14 per cent have a serious weight problem. Most people realise when they are overweight, although. If you are overweight, are you really aware of the limitations this extra weight is imposing on you? For example, if you are as much as 50 kg (8 stone) overweight you are carrying around the equivalent of a sack of coal – up and down stairs, when you're doing the shopping, when you're at work. You can imagine the extra work that your body (including your heart) is having to do to cope with this burden.

Losing weight

If you have had a heart attack you will undoubtedly have lost weight. Being ill in hospital is a very effective, if less than pleasant, way of losing weight. If you then take your recovery programme seriously, taking plenty of exercise and being careful with the food you eat, you will probably have little problem keeping your weight within an ideal range. The exercise will consume quite a few calories each day and taking regular exercise tends to boost your metabolism so you burn off more calories even in a resting state. If you heed the advice given on food in this chapter you will be eating less fat and more starch and fruit and vegetables, and this will automatically reduce the number of calories you take in; a gram of fat contains twice as many calories as a gram of starch, so if you eat less fat and more starch you very simply cut down your calorie intake.

If you are taking a lot of exercise you will also be reducing the amount of fat on your body and building up the muscles. There may in fact come a point where your weight starts to increase slightly. This is because there is no more fat to be burnt off, while muscle is still being added to your body. As muscle is heavier than fat, your weight starts to go up, although not by a huge amount.

After a heart attack your weight will be monitored carefully at your health centre, at the cardiac clinic and on the cardiac rehab programme. If it starts to go up above what you and the medical staff think is ideal, you will be encouraged to discuss with them both your exercise programme and what you eat. If this occurs, it is important that your spouse or partner and close family members are involved in the discussion and in subsequent decisions that are made about exercise and, particularly, food. As has been emphasised on many occasions in this book, the changes you need to make to prevent yourself having another heart attack are lifetime, lifelong changes. They have to involve the people you live with – if you are out on your own you will find it very difficult to stick to them. You need to have the support and cooperation of the rest of the family, particularly those who shop and cook.

To begin with, you will be encouraged to take more exercise each week or day. Perhaps it could be walking further or faster each day. You might be encouraged to go to a fitness centre once or twice a week, or to take up another activity such as swimming lengths or playing badminton. You will also receive general dietary advice along the lines set out in this chapter; problems with food will be looked at and suggestions made. This help may come from the cardiac clinic, but it is more likely to come from the cardiac rehab programme, if you are still on one, or from your GP and the staff at your health centre. The practice nurse may well run weight reduction sessions, but if you are uncomfortable about going along to such group sessions it is usually no problem to fix up personal appointments with the nurse or dietitian or GP. Make use of all these opportunities; for some people losing weight can be a real problem and if they think they have to solve it on their own it might seem insurmountable. If they know that they have the help and support of their family and various members of the healthcare team, it can seem much easier.

11 Conclusion

By the time you get to this last chapter, you should be well on your way to recovery from your heart attack or should know and understand what you have to do to ensure your recovery. The aim of this book has been to give you and those close to you as much explanation and advice as possible. The most important points to remember are:

- Don't ignore the symptoms of a heart attack. The sooner you can receive treatment, the greater the chance of minimising the damage to your heart.
- Accept the fact that you will recover but that it will take determination on your part.
- A heart attack is a life-threatening event, and affects not only the sufferer but their spouses or partners, their close family members and their close friends. All are involved in the recovery process and ideally should work together.
- The most important elements of the recovery process are stopping smoking, taking exercise and eating the right foods.
- For the recovery process to be successful, these three elements have to become an ordinary part of your life for the rest of your life.

Perhaps the last point to be emphasised – and it is a thread that has run throughout this book – is that there is a lot of help available. Sometimes it is obvious and seeks you out; sometimes it is less than obvious and you need to seek it out yourself. As well as self-determination, which will enable you seek out as much help as possible, you need an ability to accept the help that is on offer, whether it comes from your family, your friends, the health service, other people who have had heart attacks, other services, or whatever. Accepting help does not undermine you, does not make you dependent on others. Quite the opposite: it ensures that you can stand on your own feet again as swiftly as possible. Then you will be in a position to pass on the lessons you have learned, and help and support other people who have suffered heart attacks.

Glossary

ACE inhibitors A group of vasodilator drugs.

adrenaline A hormone released by the adrenal glands that prepares the body for danger or stress. Amongst other things it raises blood pressure and stimulates the heart.

aerobic exercise Steady exercise over 10 minutes or more that uses oxygen to fuel the muscles.

alpha-1 antagonists A group of vasodilator drugs.

anaerobic exercise Sudden and violent exercise over a short time that does not use oxygen to fuel the muscles.

analgesia Pain relief.

analgesics Pain-relieving drugs.

angina An acute pain caused by lack of oxygen supplied to the heart muscle; this lack of oxygen is in turn caused by atherosclerosis.

angiogram The use of a tube, inserted via the blood vessels into the heart or the coronary arteries, to inject a dye that shows up on X-ray. X-ray pictures can then be taken of the heart and coronary arteries, to see if they are diseased.

angioplasty A balloon, on the end of a fine tube inserted via the blood vessels into the coronary arteries, is inflated in an area of atherosclerosis. This stretches the narrowed area of atherosclerosis, and when the balloon is deflated and removed, the narrowed area remains wider

antiarrhythmics Drugs that keep the heart beating regularly.

anticoagulants Drugs that reduce the risk of blood clots forming.

aorta The aorta or dorsal aorta is the largest artery leaving the heart. It arches up and back from the top of the heart and descends through the abdominal cavity. It is 1 inch (2–3 cm) in diameter.

arrhythmia Any disturbance of the natural rhythm of the heart.

artery A blood vessel that carries blood from the heart to the rest of the body.

atherosclerosis The thickening and hardening of the artery walls with deposits that largely consist of cholesterol. These deposits fur up the arteries and can eventually block them.

bad cholesterol Low density lipoprotein.

beats per minute Measure of heart rate.

Benefits Agency Government agency responsible for issuing and advising on all state benefits, including statutory sick pay and incapacity benefit.

beta blockers A group of drugs used to treat high blood pressure and angina pectoris.

BMI   Body – mass index.

body – mass index A measurement calculated by dividing your weight (in kilograms) by your height squared (in metres).

Borg perceived exertion scale A scale based on your perception of the exertion involved in different exercise levels.

BPM   Beats per minute.

bypass surgery The use of a piece of blood vessel from the leg or the inside of the chest to bypass a section of diseased and narrowed coronary artery.

CABG   Coronary artery bypass graft.

calcium antagonists A group of vasodilator drugs.

cardiac catheterisation A procedure in which a fine tube is passed into the heart, either for an angiogram or angioplasty/stent.

cardiac enzymes Chemicals released when heart muscle is damaged. Testing for these enzymes is an important check on whether a heart attack has occurred.

cardiac event A heart attack.

cardiovascular accident A stroke.

catheter   A tube going into the body. Commonly refers to a tube going into the bladder, allowing you to pass urine without noticing.

CCU   Cardiac/coronary care unit.

CHD   Coronary heart disease.

cholesterol   A fatty compound essential to life. It circulates in the bloodstream in fatty complexes called lipoproteins. Cholesterol in the bloodstream is involved in forming atherosclerotic deposits.

clot   A mass of fibres and blood cells that forms a solid lump.

clot-buster   A thrombolytic drug, e.g. streptokinase.

collaterals   Tiny blood vessels that develop in parallel to existing tiny blood vessels. They might bypass diseased blood vessels, or expand the network of blood vessels to cope with demands made by a progressive exercise programme.

coronary arteries The arteries supplying blood to the heart. They are the first arteries to branch off the aorta.

coronary artery bypass graft Bypass surgery.

coronary care unit A specialised ward where heart attack patients are treated for the first 24 – 48 hours after the heart attack.

coronary heart disease Disease caused by the furring up of the coronary arteries with atherosclerotic deposits. Symptoms include breathlessness, angina and heart attacks.

CVA A cardiovascular accident, or stroke.

defibrillator A piece of equipment that delivers an electrical shock across the chest. It is used to treat ventricular fibrillation.

diabetes Disease in which the blood glucose concentration is above normal. Type I, insulin-dependent (IDDM), diabetes involves a lack of insulin; type II, non-insulin dependent (NIDDM), diabetes involves insulin acting inefficiently.

diamorphine Heroin. In the UK the drug of choice for pain relief after a heart attack.

diastole The relaxed phase of the heart's pumping action.

diastolic pressure Blood pressure during diastole.

diuretics Drugs that remove excess water from the body.

Driving and Vehicle Licensing Agency Government agency responsible for driving licences.

DVLA Driving and Vehicle Licensing Agency.

ECG Electrocardiograph.

echocardiography The use of ultrasound to provide images of the inside of the heart and an idea of blood flow in the heart.

electrocardiograph Recording of the electrical activity of the heart.

exercise ECG test An ECG taken when you are exercising on a treadmill or an exercise bike. It shows the extent of the damage to the heart after a heart attack.

fibre Indigestible plant residues that are not broken down by the process of digestion. They add bulk and roughage to the food mass in the gut.

glyceryl trinitrate The most commonly used of the nitrate drugs.

good cholesterol High density lipoprotein.

GTN Glyceryl trinitrate.

haemoglobin The chemical in the red blood cells that carries oxygen around the blood system.

Hb   Haemoglobin.

HDL   High density lipoprotein.

heart attack The degeneration of part of the heart muscle, so that it stops working. The damage is caused by furred-up coronary arteries not supplying enough oxygen and nutrients to the heart muscle.

heart rate   Number of times the heart beats per minute.

helpline   Some cardiac clinics/wards run a helpline whereby problems can be discussed with a trained cardiac nurse, who probably is involved with the rehabilitation programme.

high density lipoprotein A fatty complex that transports cholesterol from the rest of the body to the liver. It appears to remove cholesterol from atherosclerotic deposits and is referred to as 'good' cholesterol.

hypertension High blood pressure.

hypotension Low blood pressure.

incapacity benefit Benefit paid by the state if you are off sick and cannot get statutory sick pay.

infarct   Death of an area of tissue, e.g. heart muscle.

LDL   Low density lipoprotein.

lipids   A group name for fats and oils. It includes cholesterol.

lipoprotein A particle in which fats are transported in the bloodstream.

low density lipoprotein A fatty complex that transports cholesterol from the liver to the rest of the body. It appears to add cholesterol to atherosclerotic deposits and is referred to as 'bad' cholesterol.

mono-unsaturated fats Fats, largely of vegetable origin, that tend not to raise blood cholesterol levels. In some circumstances it seems they can raise HDL cholesterol levels.

myocardial infarction Death of part of the heart muscle.

myocardium The heart muscle.

nitrates   Vasodilators, specifically used to treat angina pain.

obesity   Being severely overweight.

percutaneous transluminal coronary angioplasty The full name for angioplasty.

platelets   Small particles in the blood that are involved in the clotting process. Because of this they are involved in atherosclerotic deposits.

polyunsaturated fats Fats, largely of vegetable origin, that tend not to raise blood cholesterol levels.

practice nurse A nurse who works in a heath centre, carrying out various functions that the GPs delegate to them.

PTCA Percutaneous transluminal coronary angioplasty.

repeat prescription A prescription for a specific medicine that has been prescribed before. Usually these prescriptions can be obtained simply by contacting the health centre, without the need for a doctor's appointment.

saturated fats Fats, largely of animal origin, that tend to raise blood cholesterol levels.

sickness benefit Now called incapacity benefit.

sodium chloride Cooking salt.

SSP Statutory sick pay.

starchy foods Foods rich in starch (a carbohydrate), e.g. bread, potatoes, pasta, rice, breakfast cereals, other cereals, lentils, beans and pulses.

statutory sick pay Pay from your employer when you are off sick.

stent A wire mesh-tube inserted on an angioplasty balloon into an area of atherosclerotic narrowing of the coronary arteries. When the balloon is inflated the stent expands, stretching the area of narrowing. When the balloon is deflated and removed the stent keeps the atherosclerotic area widened.

stroke Often called a cardiovascular accident, or CVA, it is an interruption to the blood supply to the brain, invariably caused by atherosclerosis.

subendocardial infarct A heart attack that only involves a portion of the heart muscle.

surgical cardiac ward Specialised ward where patients are treated after heart surgery.

systole The pumping phase of the heart's cycle.

systolic pressure Blood pressure during systole. It is greater than the diastolic pressure.

tachycardia An extremely rapid heartbeat.

thrombolytic A drug, e.g. streptokinase, that dissolves the clots that block the furred-up arteries. It reduces the chance of further damage to the heart muscle and of a subsequent heart attack in the short term. Often called a 'clot-busting' drug.

trans-fatty acids Processed fats, from a variety of origins, that behave

like saturated fats and tend to raise blood cholesterol
levels.

vasodilators Drugs that widen the arteries.

vein Blood vessel bringing blood from the rest of the body back
to the heart.

ventricular fibrillation When the electrical stimulation of the heart
goes haywire and the heart stops beating or beats very
irregularly.

water pills Diuretic drugs.

Useful addresses

Al-anon and Alateen
61 Great Dover Street
London SE1 4YF
tel 0171-403 0888

Provide help for families of problem drinkers and teenagers with drink problems. Publish a series of leaflets.

Alcohol Concern
275 Grays Inn Road London
WC1X 8FQ
tel 0171-833 3471

Ground Floor 4 Dock Chambers
Bute Street
Cardiff CF1 6AG
tel 01222 488000

Provides information, publications, advice, education and information on alcoholism.

Alcoholics Anonymous
PO Box 1
Stonebow House
Stonebow YO1 2NJ
tel 01904 644026

Baltic Chamber
50 Wellington Street
Glasgow G2 8HJ
tel 0141-226 2214

Provides help and support for problem drinkers who want to give up their drinking. The phone number for your nearest branch is in your telephone directory under Alcoholics Anonymous.

ASH (Action on Smoking and Health)
109 Gloucester Place
London W1H 3PH
tel 0171-935 3519

142 Whitchurch Road
Cardiff CF4 3NA
tel 01222 614339

8 Frederick Street
Edinburgh EH2 2HB
tel 0131-225 4725

40 Eglantine Avenue
Belfast BT9 6DX
tel 01232 663281

A charity that promotes non-smoking. Publishes a fortnightly Ash Information Bulletin, other publications, videos and details of how to run stop-smoking groups.

The British Association for Cardiac Rehabilitation
Honorary Secretary c/o British Cardiac Society
9 Fitzroy Square
London W1P 5AH
tel 0171-383 3887

The British Cardiac Society, to which the BACR is affiliated, will give you the contact address and telephone number. The BACR can give guidelines on cardiac rehabilitation and on training for those interested in setting up programmes.

The British Dietetic Association
7th Floor
Elizabeth House
22 Suffolk Street
Queensway
Birmingham B1 1LJ
tel 0121-643 5483

Gives information on diet and food.

The British Heart Foundation
14 Fitzhardinge Street
London W1H 4DH
tel 0171-935 0185

Publishes booklets on heart disease and how to reduce your risks, as well as a regular newsletter. Has lists of cardiac rehab programmes around the country and of Heartbeat self-help groups.

The British Hyperlipidaemia Association
Department of Clinical Biochemistry
Medical School
Framlington Place
Newcastle-upon-Tyne NE2 4HH

The British Lung Foundation
8 Peterborough Mews
London SW6 3BL
tel 0171-371 7704

Can give advice and help on giving up smoking.

The British Nutrition Foundation
15 Belgrave Square
London SW1X 8PG
tel 0171-235 4904

Produces a number of leaflets to do with coronary heart disease.

The British Sports Association for the Disabled
34 Osnaburgh Street
London NW1 3ND
tel 0171-383 7277

Has information on facilities available in specific areas.

The Chest, Heart and Stroke Association
65 North Castle Street
Edinburgh EH2 3LT
tel 0131-225 6963

Provides information and support for those who have suffered a heart attack.

The Consumer's Association
2 Marylebone Road
London NW1 4DF
tel 0171-486 5544

Various reports are available that compare healthy food products.

The Coronary Prevention Group
Plantation House
Suite 5/4 D&M
31/35 Fenchurch Street
London EC3M 3NN
tel 0171-626 4844

Publishes a number of booklets on coronary heart disease.

DVLA
Drivers Medical Unit
Longview Road
Morriston
Swansea SA99 1TU
tel 01792 783686

Contact this unit for information about driving after a heart attack.

The Family Heart Association
7 High Street
Kidlington OX5 2DH
tel 01865 370292

Produces various publications on coronary heart disease prevention and healthy eating.

The Flora Project for Heart Disease Prevention
24 – 8 BloomsburyWay
London WC1A 2PX
tel 0171-242 0936

Produces various publications on heart disease prevention.

The Health Education Authority
Hamilton House
Mabledon Place
London WC1H 9TX
tel 0171-383 3833

Produces a wealth of books, leaflets and other publications on all aspects of heart disease. Has regional offices, which might be of more use to you.

The Health Education Board for Scotland
Woodburn House
Canaan Lane
Edinburgh EH10 4SG
tel 0131-447 8044

Has a similar role in Scotland as the Health Education Authority in England.

**The Health Promotion
   Authority for Wales**
Brunel House
Fitzalan Road
Cardiff CF 2 1EB
tel 01222 472472

*Has a similar role in Wales as the
Health Education Authority in
England. Publishes some material
in Welsh.*

Open University
PO Box 188
Milton Keynes MK7 5DH
tel 01908 652185

A group work pack Handling
Stress *has been developed in asso-
ciation with the Health Education
Authority.*

Quit
102 Gloucester Place
London W1H 3DA
tel 0171-487 2858

*A charity helping smokers to quit.
Produces various publications.*

Sports Council
16 Upper Woburn Place
London WC1H 0QP
tel 0171-388 1277

*Publish a wide range of materials
on exercise, activity and good
health.*

Index

Page numbers in *italic* refer to the illustrations